循证医学互动教学手册(双语案例版)

Evidence-based Medicine Interaction Teaching Manual (Bilingual and Case Edition)

主编　李红梅

Editor in Chief　Li Hongmei

科学出版社

北京

内 容 简 介

互动教学法强调师生之间、生生之间的互动与交流,是一种推动教学改革、改善课堂生态的重要手段。本手册以互动教学法为主要手段对循证医学课程的课堂教学进行设计和组织,通过精心设计的案例,模拟师生之间的互动,详细展示了各种互动教学技术在不同教学内容中的应用过程,以期为循证医学或其他课程的教师提供一个可供参考的互动教学实践操作指南。

本书可供医学院校临床医学专业双语教学或全英文 MBBS 教学使用。

Interative teaching method emphasizes the interaction and communication between teachers and students and among students. It is an important means to promote teaching reform and improve classroom atmosphere. This manual designs and organizes the classroom teaching of evidence-based medicine (EBM) by means of interactive teaching method. Through elaboraely designed cases to simulate the interaction between teachers and students, the application process of various interactive techniques in different teaching contents is demonstrated in detail. Hopefully, it can provide a practical guide for teachers of EBM or other courses.

This book can be used in bilingual teaching of clinical medicine or in English MBBS teaching in medical universities.

图书在版编目(CIP)数据

循证医学互动教学手册:双语案例版 ＝ Evidence-based Medicine Interaction Teaching Manual (Bilingual and Case Edition):汉英对照 / 李红梅主编. —北京:科学出版社,2020.7
ISBN 978-7-03-065512-7

Ⅰ. ①循… Ⅱ. ①李… Ⅲ. ①循证医学-双语教学×教材-汉、英 Ⅳ. ①R499

中国版本图书馆 CIP 数据核字(2020)第 104058 号

责任编辑:闵 捷 朱 灵 / 责任校对:谭宏宇
责任印制:黄晓鸣 / 封面设计:殷 靓

科学出版社 出版
北京东黄城根北街 16 号
邮政编码:100717
http://www.sciencep.com

南京展望文化发展有限公司排版
江苏句容市排印厂印刷
科学出版社发行 各地新华书店经销

*

2020 年 7 月第 一 版 开本:B5(720×1000)
2020 年 7 月第一次印刷 印张:16
字数:294 000
定价:98.00 元
(如有印装质量问题,我社负责调换)

《循证医学互动教学手册》(双语案例版)

编委会

Evidence-based Medicine Interaction Teaching Manual
(Bilingual and Case Edition)

Editoral Board

前言

　　基于证据的诊治决策理念虽然源远流长,但循证医学真正成为一门系统的学科,并在临床推广和在大学进行教学还是近二三十年的事。其研究的内容、目的、理论和方法对于大多数的临床医生和学生来说是既熟悉又陌生的。所谓熟悉,是其研究的问题都来自临床,是医生或医学生面对患者时真正碰到的难题,其研究的目的是所有医生的目的,即为患者提供最好的诊疗;所谓陌生,指的是其理论和方法,虽然他们大部分来自现代流行病学、统计学和文献检索,但如何运用这些学科的理论和方法来解决临床决策中的问题却是全新的和颇为复杂的。因此,在学习过程中,学生容易产生轻敌和畏难两种交织的情绪。课堂也容易出现沉闷、乏味的知识授受状态。如何把课程理念转化为具体的课堂教学实践、什么样的教学形式才能充分调动学生将已有的知识与新知识相结合,使课堂真正焕发生命活力,是教师们面临的难题。

　　苏霍姆林斯基曾在《给教师的建议》一书中告诫教师:"学习——这并不是把知识从教师的头脑转移到学生的头脑里,首先是教师跟学生之间的活生生的人的相互关系。"近年来,互动教学已成为教育研究的一个热点问题,被视为推动教学改革、改善课堂教学生态的重要手段。学者们借鉴哲学、社会学的视角,或从教育理念、教育理论以及认知和心理学的角度着眼来研究互动教学法,获得了一定的理论和实践成果,但这些研究结果通常具有宏观的指导意义,而缺少与具体学科相结合的实际可操作的参照价值。广大从事一线教学的教师,尤其初次承担向临床医学学士(MBBS)学生英文教授循证医学的教师,首先课堂语言的组织是一种挑战;其次,外国学生与中国学生课堂特点的明显差异也让教师们感到气馁。本手册以互动教学法为主要手段,对循证医学课程的课堂教学进行设计和组织,通过来自教学实践的鲜活的互动案例,详细展示各种互动技术在不同教学内容中的应用过程,以期为教师提供一个可供实际操作的参照。

李红梅

2019 年 8 月于昆明

PREFACE

Although the concept of decision-making for evidence-based diagnosis and treatment has a long history, it has been nearly 20 or 30 years since evidence-based medicine became a systematic discipline and was promoted in clinical practice and teaching in universities.

The content, purpose, theories and methods of the discipline are both familiar and unfamiliar to most clinicians and students.

The so-called familiarity refers to such a fact that the research problems come from the clinic, which are the real difficulties encountered by doctors or clinical students when facing patients. The purpose of the research is the goal of all doctors, that is, to provide the best treatment for patients.

By unfamiliarity, it comes to its theories and methods. Although most of them come from modern epidemiology, statistics and literature retrieval, it is something new and rather complicated how to use the theories and methods of these disciplines to solve problems in clinical decision-making.

Therefore, in the process of learning, it's easy for the students to produce the combination of taking what they are facing lightly and fearing difficulties.

Classes are also prone to result in a boring or tedious state of giving and receiving knowledge.

It is a problem that teachers have to face how to convert the course idea into specific classroom teaching practice. It is equally the same problem and difficulty what kind of teaching form can fully mobilize the combination of students' existing knowledge and new knowledge, and make the classroom truly revitalized.

In his book *Advice to Teachers*, Suchomlinskii (B. A. Cyxomjnhcknn) gave the following advice："Learning，which is not the transfer of knowledge from the teacher's mind to the student's mind，is actually the human interaction between the teacher and the student，both as living persons".

In recent years，teaching interaction has become a hot issue in education research and is seen as an important means to promote teaching reform and improve classroom teaching ecology.

Both from the perspective of philosophy，sociology，or from the educational ideas，educational theories and cognitive and psychological perspective to study the interactive teaching method，scholars have obtained certain theoretical and practical results. These findings usually have their macro guidance effect，but it is also inevitable that they lack actual operational reference value in specific discipline combining.

For the majority of teachers engaged in front-line teaching，especially those who take the first responsibility for MBBS students' Evidence-based Medicine teaching，the organization of classroom language is a major challenge at first，and second，the obvious differences of classroom characteristics between foreign students and Chinese students also discourage the teachers.

This manual designs and organizes the classroom teaching of Evidence-based Medicine by means of interactive teaching methods. Through living interactive cases from teaching practice，the application process of various interactive teaching technologies in different teaching contents is demonstrated in detail，which is hoped to provide an operable reference for teachers.

Li Hongmei

Aug.，2019，Kunming

目 录

互动教学概述

互动教学是以互动教学技术作为手段,以师生间、生生间的意义交流为特征,充分发挥学习者在学习中的主体作用,实现主动建构并相互促进的教学形式和教学理念的总称。其表层结构是指教学过程中,师生间、生生间可观察、可记录的外在互动形式,即互动教学法;其内在的深层结构则是影响、支配互动形式的教学理念,它决定着教学互动的内涵和实质。在真实的教学活动中,教师采用的教学方法是多种多样的,如讲授法、互动教学法、参与性教学法、体验教学法、合作学习法、探究学习法等。通常是以某一方法为主,多种教学法并用为辅组织教学的。良好的教学不仅要实现不同教学方式与手段的有机组合,更重要的是基于教学理念,结合实际的教学目标与教学内容的性质,对教学过程进行精心的设计与实践。本手册以互动教学为主来组织循证医学(Evidence-based Medicine,EBM)课程的教学,目的是充分调动学生学习的积极性,从根本上焕发课堂的生命活力。

1. 互动教学法

互动教学法是基于互动教学理念,使用互动技术组织教学的一种教学方式。即在教学中采用互动并依赖于语言和非语言(如表情、动作、手势、眼神等),创造有利于学生发展的环境的教学形式。

互动教学理念认为,课堂是一个微观社会,教学是课堂中各种角色间相互作用和相互影响,并发挥其特有功能的过程。教师和学生的角色是相互平等的,教师不再是知识的权威,而是学生学习的伙伴;学生不再是知识的被动接受者,而是在教师引导下收获体验的学习主体。教学过程是师生相互作用和影响、共同发展的互动过程。与传统的填鸭式教学相比,互动教学不只是看重学习成绩,而是更加看重对学生学习习惯与学习态度的培养。

互动教学法是与学生保持持续思想交流的有效方式,它起源于被誉为哈佛大学法宝的"案例教学法",后经发展,将一系列强调师生间互动的教学方法共同归纳为互动教学法,其核心是新型师生关系的建构。它强调教学过程中教师与学生的交流与合作。通过师生之间的交流,可以解决传统教学面临的诸多问题。

它允许学生在课堂上应用他们所学的知识，也可以为马上要涉及的知识做铺垫。在课堂上应用这些方法，不仅仅从形式上让学生参与到课堂中，更能引导他们应用所学内容，并能向教师反馈学生理解的程度。

2. 互动教学技术

互动教学技术是基于某种社会心理理论或教学理念而在教学实践中逐渐形成的一些教学互动技术。这些技术被应用于不同的教学场景中，有多重益处：教师可以轻松、快速地评估学生是否真正掌握所学、是否有必要投入更多的时间；可以测量学生对于教学材料的理解过程，很多时候，评估也常常是学习材料本身的练习——通常情况下，学生们直到被要求在诸如此类的评估中使用学习材料时，才会真正地理解这些材料。此外，评估可推动交互，产生益处。这些技术常常是比较有趣的，在促进学生学习方面往往比讲课更有效。学生们从被动听讲的状态中激发起来，变得专心、投入，这也是有效学习的两个先决条件。以下所列出的是本手册中采用的互动教学技术，以及其他近年来常用的互动教学技术，部分参考自 Thomas A, Alison Morrison-Shetlar 等人的著作，部分来自近年来发表的互动教学研究论文。将它们用于 EBM 的教学中，能够很好地激发学生的参与和互动。当然，根据教学内容和教学对象，选择何种互动技术，还有赖于教师个人的教学风格和个性等因素。

（1）常用于课前调查的互动教学技术

A. 背景知识调查问卷：在引入一个新的内容时可采用问卷（多选题或简答题）了解学生的背景知识。

B. 链式笔记：教师预先分发索引卡，和一个信封，写上与学习有关的问题。（如小组讨论有用吗？）学生们在卡片上写下一个非常简短的回答，把自己的卡片投进信封，然后把信封递给下一个学生。

C. 课堂民意调查：用非正式的举手来表决。常用于对一个有争议的话题进行民意调查。

D. 空大纲：发放当天讲座的部分完成的大纲，让学生填写。用于课程开始或结束时。

E. 兴趣/知识/技能清单：评价学生对课程的兴趣和已有储备，该法可帮助教师调整其教学进度。

F. 误解调查：用于课前了解学生关于某个主题的先入之见。

G. 学习方式的自我评估：为学生准备一份调查问卷，调查他们的学习风格，在以后的课程上中就能采取与其学习风格，如视觉、听觉、触觉等学习风格相适应的教学法。

H. 学生投票：挑选一些学生(最好是志愿者)在教室里活动,就课程相关的话题对其他学生的意见进行收集,然后向全班报告结果。

(2) 常用于课前或课后复习的互动技术

A. 集体回答：教师提出一个问题(该问题的答案只需要一个词,如"是"或"否")要求全班同学一起快速作答;答对的人数将表明理解的程度。用于快速复习所学。

B. 全员身体反应(TPR)：学生用身体的姿势,如起立或坐下,来代表对教师问题的二元答案,如对或错。可用于课前或课后的快速复习。

C. 猜猜看：通过问一个有趣的问题来介绍一个新话题,这个问题很少有人知道答案(但应该引起所有人的兴趣)。在给出答案之前,接受一段时间的盲目猜测,培养好奇心。

D. 回忆—总结—提问—联系—评论：开启课程的每一环节(或每周)的方法。通过 5 个步骤来强化前一节课的内容：回忆、总结、提出余留问题、与整个课程进行联系,并评论。

E. 一分钟作文：学生们就一个特定的问题写一分钟小作文(问题可以是：你今天学到的最重要的事情是什么?)。一般用于课后。

F. 最糊涂的地方：和"一分钟作文"类似。只不过问题一般是"你今天最不清楚的是什么",而不是"你学到的最重要的是什么"。一般用于课后。

G. 建议信：让学生们就如何学好该课程给未来的学生写一封建议信。

H. 保险杠贴纸：要求学生写一个类似于标语的语句来说明课堂上的某个概念。变体为：让学生用一句话来概括整个课程。

I. 一句话总结：把某个内容总结成一个句子,该句子要包含谁、什么、何时、何地、为什么、如何等元素。

J. 单词日报：先让学生在纸上用一个单词来总结整个话题,然后再用一段话来解释该词。

K. 收获：在课堂上的一次体验/活动结束后,让学生反思他们学到了什么,为什么(它为什么重要,它的含义是什么),现在如何(如何应用它或它对你今后的影响)。

L. 小组工作评估：问卷调查关于小组活动的课堂有效性。

(3) 常用于课程中的互动技术

A. 图片提示：向学生展示一幅图片,不对其做任何说明或解释。让学生识别或解释,并评价学生的回答,或者让学生们用课堂上的术语来描述它,或者给所展示的过程和概念命名。这有助于加强学生对课堂所学内容的理解、记忆和运用,用于小组活动也很有效。在学生探索过所有的选择之前不要给出答案。

B. 思考时段：在讲授过程中，教师随时停下来，提出一个开放性的问题，让学生思考 20 秒的时间，然后再作解释。这种方法即使在不可能进行讨论的情况下，也能鼓励学生参与解决问题的过程。可以要求学生把所想到的写下来（同时教师也写一个答案），有助于确保他们专注于解决该问题。

C. 教师讲故事：教师用现实生活中的事实、模型或案例来说明一个概念、理念或原则。由于故事来源于生活实际，容易吸引学生的注意，引发学生思考，教学互动更容易展开。

D. 苏格拉底式提问：教师用一连串的追问来代替讲课。教师不断追问，而这些问题（驱动问题）始终导向最初设定的学习目标。该法以公元前 4 世纪古希腊哲学家苏格拉底的名字来命名，他曾经采用一种以通过向学生提问而促使他们发现答案为主的教学方法。他认为，经过训练的深思熟虑的提问使学者/学生们能够检省自己的想法，并能够确定这些想法的正确性。苏格拉底式提问的基础是：思维是具有结构化逻辑的，并允许潜在的思想被质疑。苏格拉底式提问是系统的、严格的、深入的，通常用于基本概念、原则、理论、争议或难题方面的教学。当教师在教学中使用苏格拉底式提问时，可以深入探究学生的思维，确定学生对给定话题、问题或主题的认知程度，培养学生提出苏格拉底问题的能力，帮助学生成为积极、独立的学习者。

E. 传递教鞭：在屏幕上展示一个综合的、复杂的或详细的图案，并将教鞭暂时递交给志愿者，让其指出关键性的特征或就其不明白的地方提出问题。

F. 讨论排：当学生自愿回答课堂上的提问时，可获得额外的学分奖励并坐在前排。这将形成一个永远准备好与教师互动的小组。

G. 手持回应卡：分发（或要求学生自己制作）标准化的卡片，学生举起不同的卡片可以作为对教师问题的回应。例如：绿色卡片代表正确，红色卡片代表错误。或者在每张卡片上写上不同的字母，代表选择题的选项。

H. 引文填空：提供一段与授课主题相关的引文，但省略了一个关键字，让学生猜它可能是什么。该法会让学生很快投入到一个话题中。

I. 大声念出来：选择一小段文字（500 字或更少）大声朗读，并要求学生在这一阶段特别注意。在大课上朗读一小段文字可以集中注意力。

（4）小组活动常用的互动技术

A. 锦标赛：将班级分成至少两组，让其就某个内容进行学习后展开竞赛，获得分数最高的为胜。比赛分好几轮，每轮比赛前都先让他们一起学习一个主题，然后进行比赛，计算分数，最后计算总分。学生的竞争冲动将会集中于他们对材料本身的投入。

B. 理解图：学生将其对一个抽象概念或想法的理解用图画表达出来。在教室里,同学们互相比较他们的图画可以消除对此概念的误解。

C. 作品展板:将学生在之前的活动中提交的图画/抽象概念进行展示,让其分组讨论并进行汇报。

D. PPT 演示:将学生分成 3～4 人的小组。学生们将注意力集中在一章或一篇文章上,并用 PPT 将这些材料在课堂上呈现。

(5) 个人活动常用的互动技术:

A. 轮流朗读:让学生一人朗读一段文字中的一句话,而不是由教师来完成整段文字或让学生各自默念。

B. 投票胶:将预先写好的话题展示在教室的粘贴板上,给学生提供一些彩色粘胶,让学生利用手中的彩色粘胶对自己同意的观点进行投票。

C. 提问优胜者:先让一些学生解答黑板上的问题。答案揭晓后,请答对了的人举手(并保持举手的动作);然后,所有其他学生都要和举手的人交谈,以便更好地理解这个问题及下次如何解决它。

D. 解题原则是什么:提出问题,学生们考虑应用什么原则来解决该问题。应帮助学生关注问题的类型而不是个别具体问题本身。事前应列出多项解题原则。

E. 对或错:分发写有一句陈述句的索引卡(每个学生一张)。一半的卡片将包含正确的陈述,另一半是错误的陈述。学生们可以用任何方式来表达他们手上的陈述属于哪一半。

F. "真实世界":让学生在课堂上讨论一个主题或概念如何在现实世界中应用或者关联。然后让学生作为课后作业写下来。变化:也可让他们把答案记录在索引卡上。

G. 概念地图:学生把关键字写在便签上,然后把这些关键字组织成流程图,结构不必复杂,只要简单地画出概念之间的联系即可。

H. 真实陈述:可用于引入一个话题或考查学生的理解程度。让每个学生对曾经讨论过的话题写出如下结构的句子:这是真实的……接下来的讨论可能会展示有时候他们掌握的知识是多么的模糊不清。

I. 反义词:教师列出一个或多个概念,学生必须想出一个反义词,然后为他们的选择提供理由。

J. 应用于本专业:用课堂最后的 15 分钟时间,让学生写一篇关于如何应用今日所学于各自专业的短文。

K. 利弊面:学生们就给定主题列出利弊面。

L. 令人钦佩的个人:学生对课程相关的某个人物进行简要的描述。学生评估自己的价值观并了解该领域的最佳实践案例。

　　M. 什么/如何/为什么概述：当分析一段文字或课文时，让学生通过写简短的笔记回答"什么/如何/为什么"的问题。

　　N. 近似类比：让学生提供类比的后半部分（例如，A 是对 B 的类比，正如 X 是对 Y 的类比）。

　　O. 问题识别任务：提供不同类型问题的案例研究，并要求学生识别问题的类型（与解决问题不同）。

　　P. 测验评价：学生们解释他们从考试中学到了什么，并评估考试的公平性、实用性和质量。

　　Q. 手指放在胸前：学生通过手指计数（从 1 到 4）来对多项选择题进行投票，他们不是把手指举到空中，而是把手指放在胸前，这样其他学生就看不到大多数学生在投票。

　　(6) 配对活动常用互动技术

　　A. 思考—讨论—分享（TPS）：学生先就某个问题进行个人思考，然后与同伴分享、比较和讨论，然后在课堂上发言。可用于配对活动，也可用于小组活动。

　　B. 配对—分享—重复（PSR）：配对、分享后，请学生寻找新伙伴，并向新伙伴汇报原先伙伴的经验。

　　C. 教师和学生：学生们先就上一次作业的要点进行思考，然后两两配对，分饰教师和学生的角色。其中教师的任务是概述要点，而学生的任务是把教师提到的要点划掉，但要找出 2～3 个被教师遗漏的要点。

　　D. 聪慧的另一个：个人经头脑风暴或一些富于创造性的活动后，与同伴一起分享思考或活动的结果。然后邀请一些认为其同伴的工作甚有趣味或值得分享的志愿者来说一说他们的同伴。学生们有时更愿意在全班面前分享自己同学的工作，而不是他们自己的工作。

　　E. 强迫辩论：学生两人一组进行辩论，但必须捍卫与他们个人观点相反的一方的观点。也可采取半个班的学生持一种立场，另一半持相反立场。他们站成一排，面对着对方。每个学生只能发言一次，以便双方学生都能参与讨论。

　　F. 同伴评议写作任务：给学生布置一个写作任务，鼓励他们与同伴交换草稿。合作伙伴阅读草稿后写一篇三段文回复：第一段概述文章的优点，第二段讨论文章存在的问题，第三段描述如果该文是自己的文章，将会在修改中注意的问题。

　　G. 精神分析：学生们两人一组配对，就最近的一个学习单元互相采访。不过，谈话的重点是分析材料而不是死记硬背。采访问题的范例如：你能给我描述一下你今天想分析的话题吗？ 在这个话题之前，你的态度/信念是什么？ 在了解了这个话题之后，你的态度/信念是如何改变的？ 根据你对这个话题的了解，你的行动/决定将如何改变？你对他人/事件的看法有何变化。

（7）分组技术

A. 拼图（小组专家）：指定一人为专家，给每个小组一个不同的讨论主题。然后，除专家外的其余学生重新分组，或者专家与其余学生一起重新分组。专家必须承担起介绍主题的责任。

B. 题板轮换：将学生按组分配到事先设置好的题板前（最好是 4 个或更多），每个题板上都有一个讨论的主题/问题。每个小组写完答案后，转到下一块题板上，并在前一组答案下面写下他们的答案，以此类推。

C. 传递问题：将学生分组。分配给第一组学生 1 个案例或 1 个问题，让他们找出（并写下）解决问题或分析案例的第一步（3 分钟），然后把问题传递给下一组，并让下一组的学生找出（并写下）解决问题的下一步，直到所有组都贡献了自己的力量。

D. 分层蛋糕讨论：每一桌/小组花几分钟完成相同的一件任务，然后向全班进行一次全体汇报。换新的任务后再重复一次。

E. 演讲反应：将课堂分成四个组：提问者（必须提出与材料相关的两个问题），举例者（提供应用实例），有分歧的思考者（必须提出不同意演讲的某些观点）和同意者（解释他们同意或认为有用的观点）。讨论后，每组分别向全班同学汇报。

F. 快速分组：通过生日快速将学生分为两个大致相同的组。例如，如果生日是奇数，做任务 X；如果生日是偶数，做任务 Y。其他快速分组法还包括按男性或女性、出生月份、身高是奇数或偶数分。

G. 波浪：可以将学生进行有效分组，同时也可以让学生们进行课间放松。请同学们从 1 到 n 依次报数（n 为所需组数），记住自己的号码。接着，教师从 1 到 n 依次叫号，相同号码的同学依次起立并高举双臂，同时叫出自己的号码，在另一组号码起立时坐下，起起伏伏像波浪一样。相同号码的同学成为一个小组。

（8）破冰技术

A. 推销：让学生两两配对，并通过观察了解对方不被人注意的特点。然后把他的同伴介绍给全班。教师可以利用这段时间记录学生的大致座位和名字。

B. 与名人擦肩：让学生介绍他们最近与某个名人的亲密接触的故事，即使这是一个发生在朋友或亲戚身上的故事。

C. 名字游戏：学生们以 8～10 人为一组，每次一名学生，用押头韵的方式介绍自己的名字。例如，我在跳，詹姆斯！如果能配合相应的动作最好。介绍依次进行，每次喊出前一名学生的韵、名字配合相应动作，并把自己的韵、名字、动作加在后面，直到最后一名学生说出所有人的名字和做出所有动作。

D. 排舞:学生们根据他们对一个有争议的话题的认同程度来排队,强烈认同的排成一排,强烈反对的排成一排。

E. 姓名标签三人组:在有颜色的标签上写下自己的名字,颜色相同的成为一组,然后自我介绍。

F. 速滑:让学生排成一个圈,学生依次像奥林匹克速滑运动一样,在圆圈里快速移动,同时对自己作简短的描述(我是尼泊尔人,我不吃牛肉,我喜欢古典音乐),然后回到原地。

(9) 角色扮演

A. 角色扮演:为学生分配角色,让其在家里自行研究和排演,然后在课堂上表演。观察者进行评论和提问。

B. 角色互换:教师扮演学生,就教过的内容进行提问。全体学生扮演教师,必须回答问题。该法对完成考试复习/准备工作很有效。

C. 门诊角色扮演:将课堂分成不同的角色(包括医生、上级医生、患者、患者家属等)来讨论有争议的话题。

D. 新闻发布会:邀请一名客座演讲者,像新闻发布会一样进行授课,并准备一些发言稿,然后回答听众的问题。

E. 分析备忘录:将问题分析写下来,扮演雇主或客户的角色。

(10) 头脑风暴法

A. 小组概念地图:在教室里的桌子上放上大张的招贴纸,每张上面只有一个中心节点。参与者可以在教室里任意走动,在每个招贴纸上添加子节点,直到海报满为止。

B. 在黑板上进行头脑风暴:学生们大声说出与将要介绍的主题相关的概念和术语;教师把它们写在黑板上。如果可能,将学生们的答案进行分组记录。该法用以衡量既存知识以让学生将注意力集中在某一主题上。

C. 头脑风暴树:在黑板上进行头脑风暴时,圈出主要的概念,对这些特定的词进行头脑风暴。结果就像一棵树向外开枝散叶。

D. 环形头脑风暴:组织学生一起讨论一个问题,然后让其花几分钟记笔记。一个人开始头脑风暴列表,并把它传递给右边的学生,然后这个学生将自己的内容添加上去,并再次传递。

3. 在循证医学教学中运用互动教学策略

循证医学是遵循最佳医学研究证据、结合医生临床经验和患者的意愿对患者进行科学诊治的一门方法学。其目的在于不断提高临床医疗质量和医学人才的素质,并促进医学的发展,是医生进行终身学习、更新医学知识的一门很重要的课程,也是一门实践性很强的课程。如何改变传统的教师在上、学生在下的灌输方式,改变教师单向输出、学生被动学习的教学常态,如何通过运用一定的互动技术,加强师生和生生互动,促进学生理解和知识内化,是教师们常常思考的问题。本书可被看作是一次为推动循证医学教学改革、改善课堂教学生态的重要尝试。

目前国内有关循证医学和留学生教学的研究较少,且主要集中在两方面:将循证医学的理念引入某一医学课程的教学中;将问题驱动教学法(PBL)用在留学生循证医学教学中。有关具体的互动教学技术在循证医学教学中的运用的研究则比较少。事实上,教师不一定要从形式上选择某一种特定的方法,也不一定用到上面提到的互动技术。因为教师更应该关注的是提供更多的交互式教学机会。有学者对课堂互动有效性的设计策略提出了三条建议:① 活动目标必须有明确的指向性,即课堂互动活动的设计必须直接指向预设的具体教学目标,活动的程序紧紧围绕这个教学目标展开。② 课堂互动活动的设计必须能够引起学生的参与动机。③ 在课堂互动活动形成和结构设计上,可采取简约性策略,即活动的过程要简略清晰,活动形式要简约质朴,课堂互动的频率要简约适当。遵循上述原则进行循证医学的互动策略设计大抵是不错的。

4. 如何运用本手册

本手册共 11 章,除绪论外,每章均由三部分构成:第一部分是教学要求,第二部分是教学设计,第三部分是教学内容。读者可通过第一部分"教学要求",了解本章教学目的、学习目标、主要采用的教学方法和为学生提供的阅读材料。第二部分为"教学设计",用表格的形式列出本章教学的教学内容、顺序、采用的互动策略和时间分配。第三部分为"教学内容",按顺序描述教学内容。其中,互动活动部分通过模拟师生间的互动,详细展示了师生、生生互动的过程,目的是为循证医学的教师提供一个可供参考的实践操作指导,为本手册的一大特点。循证医学具体的内容部分则较为简略,如有必要,读者可参看其他循证医学相关著作或教材。

李红梅

Introduction

Overview of Interactive Teaching

Interactive teaching is the overall description of teaching forms and teaching concept using interactive teaching techniques as a means characterized by the meaningful communication between teachers and students, and among students. Its purpose is to seize the main role of learners in learning, so as to realize active construction and mutual promotion. Its surface structure refers to the external interactive forms that can be observed and recorded between teachers and students, and among students in the teaching process, that is, the interactive teaching method. Its inner deep structure is the teaching concept that influences and dominates the forms of interaction, which determines the connotation and essence of teaching. In practical teaching activities, teachers adopt a variety of teaching methods, such as lectures, interactive teaching method, participatory teaching method, experiential teaching method, cooperative learning method, inquiry learning method, etc., and the teaching activities are usually based on a main method while a variety of other methods are equally used as auxiliary teaching. A good teaching should not only achieve the integral combination of different teaching methods and means, but more importantly, also design and practice teaching methods which elaborately integrate with the actual teaching objectives and the nature of teaching contents based on a teaching concept. This manual organizes the teaching process of evidence-based medicine mainly by means of interactive teaching. Its purpose is to fully mobilize the students' enthusiasm for learning and fundamentally revitalize the vigor of the classroom.

1. Interactive teaching method

Interactive teaching method is a kind of teaching method based on the concept of interactive teaching in which interactions between teachers and students are involved, that is, it adopts interactive techniques in teaching and relies on language and non-language (such as facial expressions, movements, gestures, eyes, etc.) to create an environment conducive to the development of students.

The concept of interactive teaching holds that a classroom is a micro-society and teaching is a process in which various roles interact and influence each other and give play to their unique functions. The roles of a teacher and the students are equal to each other. A teacher is no longer the authority of knowledge, but the partner of student learning. Students are no longer passive recipients of knowledge, but learning subjects who gain experience under the guidance of teachers. The teaching process is the interactive process of teacher-student interaction, influence and mutual development. Compared with the traditional spoon-feed teaching, the emphasis is no longer on academic achievement, but more on the cultivation of students' learning habits and attitudes.

Interactive teaching method is an effective way to maintain continuous ideological communication with students. It originated from the "case teaching method" which is praised as the magic weapon of Harvard University. With the development, a series of teaching ways that emphasize the interaction between teachers and students are collectively generalized as interactive teaching method. It emphasizes the communication and cooperation between teachers and students in the teaching process. The communication between teachers and students can solve many problems faced by traditional teaching. It allows students to apply what they've learned in class, and it also prepares them for what they're about to learn. The application of these methods in the classroom not only enables students to participate formally in the classroom, but also guides them to apply what they have learned, and to feed back the degree of their understanding to the teacher.

2. Interactive techniques

Interactive techniques are kinds of interactive teaching models based on some social psychological theory or teaching idea, which are gradually developed in teaching practice. These techniques can be applied in different teaching situations. They have multiple benefits: the instructor can easily and quickly assess if students have really mastered the material or if it is necessary to dedicate more time to them. They can also be used to measure the understanding process of students to teaching materials. In many cases, assessing is also the practice requirement of the material itself — often, students do not actually master the material until they are asked to make use of it in assessments. Furthermore, the very nature of these assessments drives interactivity and brings several benefits. These techniques are often perceived as fun; they are frequently more effective than lectures at enabling student to learn. Students are revived from the passivity of merely listening to a lecture and instead, get more attentive and engaged, and these are two prerequisites for effective learning.

The interactive techniques listed below are those adapted in this manual and some are commonly used in recent years. They are in part from works by Thomas A, Alison Morrison-Shetlar and others, and partly from the interactive teaching research papers published in recent years. Using them in the teaching of EBM will be able to stimulate students' participation and interaction. Of course, according to the teaching contents and teaching objectives, choose what kind of interactive technology will also depend on factors such as teachers' personal teaching style and personality.

（1）Interactive techniques used in pre-class surveys

A. Background knowledge probe: Use questionnaire（multi-choice or short answer）when introducing a new topic.

B. Chain notes: A teacher distributes index cards and an envelope, on which a question related to the learning is written.（i.e., are the group discussions useful?）A student writes down a very brief answer on his card, and put the card in the envelope, and passes the envelope to the next student.

C. Classroom opinion polls: Informal hand-raising is used to poll on a controversial topic.

D. Empty Outlines: A partially completed outline of today's lecture is distributed to ask students to fill it in. It is used at the start or at the end of the classes.

E. Interest/knowledge/skills checklist: It is used to assess students' interest in the course and their preparation for it. It can help adjust the teaching agenda.

F. Misconception check: It is used to learn about students' preconceptions about certain topic, which is useful for starting new chapters.

G. Self-assessment of learning methods: A questionnaire is prepared for students, which is used to know about what kind of learning style they use, so that the course can match them well in visual, aural, and tactile styles.

H. Student polling: Some students (prefer volunteers) are selected to work around the classroom, collecting the opinions of other students on topics relevant to the course, and then report the results to the class.

(2) Interactive techniques used in pre-class or post-class review

A. Choral response: The teacher asks the class to quickly answer a question that requires only one word, such as "yes" or "no". The number of correct answers will indicate the degree of understanding. It is used for quick review.

B. Total physical response (TPR): Students use body gestures, such as standing up/sitting down, to indicate their binary answers such as true or false to the teacher's questions. It can be used for quick review before or after class.

C. Make them guess: Introduce a new subject by asking an intriguing question, to which few will know the answer (but should interest all of them). Blind guessing is acceptable for a while before giving the answer so that curiosity may be built.

D. Recall-summarize-question-connect-comment: This method of starting each session (or each week) has five steps to reinforce the previous session's material: recall it, summarize it, phrase a remaining question, connect it to the class as a whole, and comment on that class session.

E. One-minute papers: Students write for one minute on a specific question. (Which might be generalized to — what was the most important thing you learned today?) Best used at the end of the class session.

F. Muddiest point: Like one-minute paper, but instead, it is used for the most confusing point. Best used at the end of the class session.

G. Advice letter: Students write a letter of advice to future students on how to be successful students in that course.

H. Bumper stickers: Ask students to write a slogan-like bumper sticker to illustrate a particular concept from lecture. Variation: Ask them to sum up the entire course in one sentence.

I. One-sentence summary: Summarize the topic into one sentence that incorporates who/what/when/where/why/how creatively.

J. Word journal: First, summarize the entire topic on paper with a single word. Then use a paragraph to explain the chosen word.

K. Harvesting: After an experience/activity in class, ask students to reflect on — what they learned, why (why it is important, what its implications are), how (how to apply it now or how it affects you in the future).

L. Group-work evaluations: Questionnaires asking how effective groupwork has been in the class.

(3) Interactive techniques used in process of the class

A. Picture prompt: Show students an image with no explanation, and ask them to identify or explain it, and justify their answers. Or ask students to write about it using terms from lecture, or to name the processes and concepts shown before. It is helpful to strengthen students' understanding, memory and application of what they have learned in class. It also works well in a group activity. Do not give the answer until they have explored all options first.

B. Think break: In the teaching process, the teacher stops at any time, ask an open-ended question, and then allow 20 seconds for students to think about the question before the teacher goes on to explain it. This technique encourages students to take part in the problem-solving process even when discussion isn't feasible. Having students write down what they have in mind (while teacher writes an answer also) helps assure that they will in fact work on the problem.

C. Instructor storytelling: Teacher illustrates a concept, idea, or principle with a real-life application, model, or case. As the story comes from the reality of life, it is easy to attract students' attention, inspire their thinking and make the teaching interaction easier to carry out.

D. Socratic questioning: The teacher replaces lecture by peppering students with questions, always asking the next question in a way that guides the conversation toward a learning outcome (or major driving question) that was desired from the beginning, which was named after Socrates, who was a philosopher in 4th century BC. Socrates utilized an educational method that focused on discovering answers by asking questions from his students. Socrates believed that "the disciplined practice of thoughtful questioning enables the scholar/student to examine ideas and be able to determine the validity of those ideas". Socratic questioning is based on the foundation that thinking has structured logic, and allows underlying thoughts to be questioned. Socratic questioning is systematic, disciplined and deep, so it is usually used to introduce fundamental concepts, principles, theories, issues or problems. When teachers use Socratic questioning in teaching, they may deeply probe student thinking, to determine the extent of students' knowledge on a given topic, issue or subject, to foster students' abilities to give Socratic questions, to help students become active and independent learners.

E. Pass the pointer: Display a comprehensive, complex, or detailed pattern on a screen and temporarily hand the pointer to the volunteer who may points out key features or asks questions about what he doesn't understand.

F. Discussion row: Students take turns sitting in a front row. They can earn extra credit as individuals when they volunteer to answer questions posed in class; this provides a group that will always be prepared and interact with teacher.

G. Hand-held response cards: Distribute standardized cards (or ask students to make) that can be held aloft as visual responses to teacher's questions. For example, a green card for being true, a red card for being false. Or handwrite a giant letter on each card to use in multiple choice questions.

H. Quote minus one: Provide a quote relevant to your topic but leave out a crucial word and ask students to guess what it might be. This engages them quickly in a topic and makes them feel invested.

I. Read aloud: Choose a small text (500 words or less) to read aloud, and ask students to pay particular attention during this phase of lecture. A small text which is read orally in a larger lecture can focus attention.

(4) Interactive techniques commonly used for group activities

A. Tournament: Divide the class into at least two groups and announce a competition in which the group that gets higher points wins. Let students study a topic together and then give that quiz before the points are given. After each round, let them study the next topic before quizzing again. The points should be carried over from round to round. The student impulse for competition will focus themselves on their engagement in the material itself.

B. Drawing for understanding: Students illustrate an abstract concept or idea. Comparing their drawings can clear up misconceptions.

C. Board of artwork: Display publicly the collected drawings/abstract concepts that students turned in for a previous activity and create an opportunity for discussion and debrief.

D. Power Point (PPT) presentation: Devide students into groups of three or four. Students focus their attention on a chapter or article and present this material to the class using Power Point.

(5) Interactive techniques commonly used for personal activities

A. Turn-taking reading: Instead of reading a paragraph by the teacher (or leaving the students to read it silently), let one student read one sentence, then someone else — anyone — continue with the next sentence.

B. Voting dots: Provide students with colored dot stickers and ask them to vote for statements they agree to most. Use up their limited dot supply on the written topics displayed around the room on poster boards.

C. Ask the winner: Ask students to silently solve a problem on the board. After revealing the answer, instruct those who got it right to raise their hands (and keep them raised); then, all other students are to talk to someone with a raised hand to better understand the question and how to solve it next time.

D. What's the principle: After putting forward a problem, students assess what principles to apply in order to solve it. Helps from the teacher should focus on problem types rather than an individual specific problem. Principle(s) should be listed out.

E. True or false: Distribute index cards (one to each student) on which a statement is written. Half of the cards contain statements that are true, half false. Students decide whether theirs is one of the true statements or not, using whatever means they desire.

F. "Real-world": Have students discuss in class how a topic or concept relates to a real-world application or product. Then have students write about this topic for homework. Variation: ask them to record their answers on index cards.

G. Concept mapping: Students write keywords onto sticky notes and then organize them into a flowchart, which could be less structured. Students simply draw the connections among concepts.

H. Truth statements: Either to introduce a topic or check comprehension. Ask each student to list out "It is true that ..." statements on the topic being discussed. The ensuing discussion might illustrate how ambiguous knowledge they have might be sometimes.

I. Opposites: Teacher lists out one or more concepts, for which students must come up with an antonym, and then defend their choice.

J. Application to professional field: During the last 15 minutes of class, ask students to write a short article about how what they learn today applies to their professional field.

K. Pro and con grid: Students list out the pros and cons for a given subject.

L. Profiles of admirable individuals: Students write a brief profile of an individual in a field related to the course. Students assess their own values and learn best practices for this field.

M. What/how/why outlines: Write brief notes answering the what/how/why questions while analyzing a message or text.

N. Approximate analogies: Students provide the second half of an analogy (A is to B as X is to Y).

O. Problem recognition tasks: Offer case studies with different types of problems and ask students to identify the type of problem (which is different from solving it).

P. Exam evaluations: Students explain what they are learning from the tests, and evaluate the fairness, usefulness, and quality of tests.

Q. Fingers on chest: Students vote on multiple choice questions by showing a finger count (1 through 4). Rather than raise them into the air, they hold their fingers before their chests so other students don't see what the majority is voting.

（6）Interactive techniques commonly used in matching activities

A. Think-pair-share（TPS）：A student shares and compares possible answers to a question with a partner before addressing the larger class. It can be used for pairing activities or group activities.

B. Pair-share-repeat（PSR）：After a pair-share experience, ask a student to get a new partner and debrief the wisdom of the old partnership to this new partner.

C. Teacher and student：Students individually brainstorm the main points of the last homework, then assign roles of teacher and student to pairs. The teacher's job is to sketch the main points, while the student's job is to cross off points on his list as they are mentioned, but come up with 2 - 3 ones missed by the teacher.

D. Wisdom of another：After any individual brainstorm or creative activity, the students, together with their partners, share their results. Then, ask the volunteers of the students who find their partners' work interesting or exemplary to talk about their partners. Students are sometimes more willing to share the work of fellow students than their own work.

E. Forced debate：Students debate in pairs, but must defend the opposite side of their personal opinion. Variation：half the class take one position, half the other. They line up and face each other. Each student may only speak once, so that all students on both sides can engage the issue.

F. Peer review writing task：Assign students with a writing assignments, and encourage them to exchange drafts with partner. The partner reads the essay and writes a three-paragraph response：the first paragraph outlines the strengths of the essay, the second paragraph discusses the essay's problems, and the third paragraph is a description of what the partner would focus on in revision, if it were his/her essay.

G. Psychoanalysis：Students get into pairs and interview one another about a recent learning unit. The focus, however, is upon analysis of the material rather than rote memorization. Sample Interview Questions：Can you describe to me the topic that you would like to analyze today? What were your attitudes/beliefs before this topic? How did your attitudes/beliefs change after learning about this topic? How have your actions/decisions altered based on your learning of this topic? How have your perceptions of others/events been changed?

(7) Grouping techniques

A. Jigsaw (group experts): Each group, with an appointed expert, is given a different topic. Then, in addition to the expert, the rest of the students regrouped, or regrouped with the expert. The expert must take on the task of introducing the topic.

B. Board rotation: Assign groups of students to each of the boards you have set up in the room (four or more works best), and assign one topic/question per board. After each group writes an answer, they rotate to the next board and write their answer below the first, and so on around the room.

C. Pass the problem: Divide students into groups. Give the first group a case or a problem and ask them to identify (and write down) the first step in solving the problem or analyzing the case (3 minutes). Pass the problem on to the next group and have them identify (and write down) the next step. Continue until all groups have contributed.

D. Layered cake discussion: Every table/group works on the same task for a few minutes, then there's a plenary debrief for the whole class, and finally repeat with a new topic to be discussed in the groups.

E. Lecture reaction: Divide the class into four groups after a lecture: questioners (must ask two questions related to the material), example givers (provide applications), divergent thinkers (must disagree with some points of the lecture), and agrees (explain which points they agreed with or found helpful). After discussion, brief the whole class.

F. Quick division: Divide your class into two roughly equal segments for simultaneous, parallel tasks by invoking their date of birth: if your birthday falls on an odd-numbered day, do task X … if your birthday is even, do task Y. Other variations include males and females, months of birth, odd or even inches in their height.

G. Wave: Wave can effetively groups students and let students relax between classes as well. Ask students to call out a number form 1 to n one by one and remember their own numbers (n is the needed number of groups). Then the teacher calls from 1 to n in turn, the students of the same number stand up in turn and raise their arms, at the same time call out their own numbers, sit down when the other group of numbers stand up, raise and fall like waves. Students with same number will be in a group.

(8) Icebreakers

A. Marketing: Students partner up and are tasked with learning one thing about the other person that is not obvious by looking at them. Then, they introduce their partner to the larger class. Teachers can use this time to record a rough seating chart of the students and begin to learn their names.

B. Brush with fame: Students relate their closest encounter with someone famous, even if it has to be a story about something that happened to a friend or relative.

C. Name game: Students form circles in groups of 8 - 10 and one at a time states his name with an alliterative action — I'm Jumping James! Optimally, they should perform the action as well. They proceed around the circle, stating names and performing the actions, adding names one at a time, until the last person in the circle will have to say everyone's name and perform all the actions.

D. Line dance: Students line up according to their level of agreement on a controversial subject: strong agreement on one side, strong disagreement on the other.

E. Name tag trio: Color code name tags and ask people to form groups of three made up of people with nametags of the same color, then introduce themselves.

F. Speed skating: Like the Olympic sport that moves in a circle rapidly, line up students in a circle and step forward one at a time to say a quick personal statement (I am Nepalese, I don't eat beef, I love classical music.) and then step back into position.

(9) Role-play

A. Role-playing: Assign students roles to study and rehearse at home, then act them out in class. Observers comment and ask questions.

B. Role reversal: Teacher acts as a student and asks questions about what has been taught. All the students acting as teachers must answer the questions. This method is very effective in preparing for exams.

C. Out-patient role-play: Divide the class into various roles (including a doctor, superior doctor, patient, family members of patient, etc.) to deliberate on a controversial subject.

D. Press conference: Invite a guest speaker and run the class like a press conference, with a few prepared remarks and then answer questions from the audience.

E. Analytic memo: Write a one-page analysis of an issue, playing the roles of an employer or client.

(10) Brainstorming

A. Group concept mapping: Place large poster boards on tables around the room, each with only one central node. Participants can walk around the classroom, adding sub-nodes to each poster until they are full.

B. Brainstorming on the board: Students speak out concepts and terms related to a topic to be introduced. The teacher writes them on the board. If possible, group the responses as they are recorded. The method is used to measure existing knowledge to get students to focus on a particular topic.

C. Brainstorming tree: As you brainstorm on the blackboard, circle the main concepts and brainstorm the specific words. The result is like a tree spreading its branches.

D. Brainstorming in a circle: Group students to discuss an issue together, and then spend a few minutes jotting down individual notes. One person starts a brainstorming list and passes it to the student to the right, who then adds to the list and passes it along again.

3. Using interactive techniques in EBM

EBM is a methodology for the scientific diagnosis and treatment of patients according to the best medical research evidence, combined with doctors' clinical experience and patients' wishes. Its aim is to improve the quality of clinical medical treatment and medical talents and to promote the development of medicine. It is a very important course for doctors to study and update medical knowledge for lifelong, and also a practical one. To change the traditional way of instilling, in which teachers tend to give and students are accustomed to taking, to change the one-way output norm of teaching and learning, to use interactive technology to strengthen the interaction between students and teachers, to promote students' understanding and knowledge internalization, this book might be regarded as an important attempt to promote the reform of evidence-based medicine teaching and improve the ecology of classroom teaching.

At present, researches on EBM teaching and foreign students' teaching in China remain to be improved. They mainly focus on two aspects: introducing the concept of EBM into the teaching of a medical course; using Problem-Based Learning（PBL）teaching method in EBM class for overseas students. There are relatively fewer researches on the application of specific interactive teaching techniques in evidence-based medicine teaching. In fact, teachers don't necessarily need to choose a particular method, nor do they need to use the interactive techniques mentioned above. Teachers should only pay attention to providing more interaction opportunities. A scholar put forward three suggestions to the design of the effectiveness of classroom interaction strategy：① The target must have a clear direction, namely the design of the interactive classroom activities must be directly pointed to a specific teaching goal, and the activity program must be centered on the teaching target. ② The design of classroom interaction activities must be able to cause the students' participation motivation. ③ In the formation and structural design of classroom interactive activities, the strategy of simplicity may be adopted. That is, the process of the activity should be brief and clear; the form of the activity should be simple and plain; the frequency of classroom interaction should be simple and appropriate. It is generally good to design interactive strategy in accordance with the above principles.

4. How to use this manual

This manual has 11 chapters. Each chapter consists of three parts: part I is teaching requirements, part Ⅱ is teaching design, and part Ⅲ is teaching contents. In Part Ⅰ, "teaching requirements", readers can acquire the objectives of teaching and learning, the primary teaching methods and the reading materials for students. In Part Ⅱ, "teaching design", the teaching contents, sequence, interactive strategy and time allocation are listed in tabular form. In Part Ⅲ, "teaching contents", which are described in order. The "interactive activity" part, by simulating the interaction between teachers and students, shows the interactive process between teachers and students, and among students, both in detail. The purpose is to provide EBM teachers with a reference to practice and operation guidance, which is a major feature of this manual. The contents of evidence-based medicine in this manual is relatively simple, and readers can refer to EBM books or textbooks, if necessary.

Li Hongmei

第 1 章

循证医学概述

第一部分 教 学 要 求

此教学环节首先介绍循证医学(EBM)课程的概况、评价方法、学习方法和对学生的要求。其次介绍了循证医学——这一临床决策新模式的概念及其三个基本要素。着重让学生通过阅读经典文献及互动环节,掌握什么是循证医学而什么不是,以及实践循证医学的优势和劣势。

1. 教学目的

讨论循证医学的概念、三要素、实践循证医学的必要性和可行性,以及实践循证医学的利弊。

2. 学习目标

通过此环节的学习,学生能够:
(1) 给循证医学下定义。
(2) 描述循证医学三要素。
(3) 列出实践循证医学的优势。
(4) 列出实践循证医学的劣势。

3. 教学方法

此环节采用互动教学法、讲授法及 PPT 演示,互动教学技术包括推销、背景知识调查、思考时段、波浪和头脑风暴法。

4. 阅读材料

(1) Sackett D L, et al. Evidence based medicine: what it is and what it isn't. BMJ, 1996, 3(12): 12.

(2) Guyatt G, Rennie D. User's guide to the medical literature:

essentials of evidence-based clinical practice. Chicago：AMA Pewaa，2001：3 - 22.

（3）Volk R J，Llewellyn-Thomas H，Stacey D，et al. Ten years of the International Patient Decision Aid Standards Collaboration：evolution of the core dimensions for assessing the quality of patient decision aids. Bmc Medical Informatics & Decision Making，2013，13 Suppl 2(S2)：S1.

第二部分　教学设计——2 课时（80 分钟）

"循证医学概述"教学设计表

序号	内　容	互动技术/教学技术	描　　　　述	时间（分钟）
1	师生互相介绍	互动 1.1：推销	向学生介绍教学团队成员，并让学生把自己介绍给同桌，并请几名学生向全班介绍其同桌	10
2	课前调查	互动 1.2：背景知识调查	分发和回收"课前调查问卷"（问卷见附录Ⅰ）	10
3	课程概述及考核标准	PPT 演示	通过 PPT 简要介绍本课程研究的内容和安排，本课程考核标准和要求	10
4	学习方法介绍	PPT 演示	学生做好课前准备及课后复习： 1. 向学生强调课前阅读相关文献的重要性。这些文献已经上传至网络课程（演示登录网络课程的方法） 2. 向学生强调积极参与互动的重要性 3. 介绍 KWL 表。请学生课后必须完成 KWL 表（可作为学习日记），并在下一节课进行讨论和分享（KWL 表见附录Ⅱ）	10
5	循证医学简介	互动 1.3：思考时段 PPT 演示	向学生展示一些没有确定答案的临床问题，请学生思考如果自己是临床医生，将如何寻找答案，从而引出"循证医学"概念	20
6	关于循证医学的讨论	互动 1.4：波浪和头脑风暴法	采用波浪互动技术将学生分为 5 人小组，要求学生阅读 Sackett D L 的文献，并讨论实践循证医学的优劣势，最后完成小组任务：关于实践循证医学优劣势的思维导图	20

第三部分　教学内容

1. 师生介绍

教师向学生介绍承担本课程的教师队伍，请学生向其同桌介绍自己，并邀请两三名学生向全班"推销"他们的同桌。

互动 1.1： 推销

（此为第一节课，通过此互动活动，可以活跃气氛，同时培养学生聆听他人、记忆并加工再现的能力。）

教师： 各位已认识我们的教学团队了，现在我请你们用 3 分钟的时间向自己的同桌介绍自己，可以是姓名、来自哪里、你的家庭、爱好、拿手的技艺等，稍后我会邀请几名学生向全班同学推销自己的同桌。

……时间到。有谁愿意来"推销"一下自己的同桌呢？好的，请这位同学先来。

学生 1： 我旁边的这位，是一个非常酷的家伙，他来自斯里兰卡，是家里的老二，他家有 5 个兄弟姐妹，他非常喜欢吃中国菜，有时会自己做菜……

教师： 你吃过他做的菜吗？味道如何？很好呀？很好！还有吗？没有啦，好的，下一位

学生 2： 我这位同桌叫阿沙，来自印度，她很会唱歌，如果她不是学医的话，肯定会是个超级巨星。

教师： 哦，真的吗？我们能请这位明星为我们表演一下吗？

……

2. 课前问卷调查

采用一份针对本课程设计的问卷对学生的学习态度和学习背景进行调查。该问卷将在课前和课程结束后调查（问卷见附录Ⅰ）。

互动 1.2： 背景知识调查

教师： 现在，我需要请两位志愿者帮助我分发问卷。

这份问卷主要了解同学们学习的习惯和需求，你的选择不会对课程的成绩产生任何影响，请各位按自己真实的情况填写。有些是单选题，有些题则可以多选。

学生：我需要填写姓名吗？

教师：不需要填写。请在 10 分钟内完成

（采用问卷调查的方式可以很好地获得学生的反馈信息。）

3. 课程概述

本课程包括 10 个教学环节，提供大家关于循证医学的重要知识和技能：
（1）绪论。
（2）临床问题的提出。
（3）证据类型和分级。
（4）临床证据的检索。
（5）临床实践中的患者价值观。
（6）治疗性研究证据的评价。
（7）病因学研究证据的评价。
（8）诊断性研究证据的评价。
（9）预后性研究证据的评价。
（10）系统评价和 Meta 分析。

学生成绩由三部分构成：完成三次作业，共 45 分，每次作业占 15%；考勤和课堂表现占 10%；期末笔试占 45%。

4. 学习方法

学生必须在课前做好预习及课后做好复习，具体要求：
（1）课前完成阅读任务。要求阅读的文献已放在网络课程中，学生自行下载打印（介绍登录网络课程的方法）。
（2）积极参与课堂互动。
（3）课后完成 KWL 表（KWL 表将来可作为你们的学习日志以供复习），并在下一节课进行讨论和分享（KWL 表见附录Ⅱ）。

5. 循证医学简介

互动 1.3：思考时段

教师：在真实的临床实践中，医生每天都会遇到很多的问题，但据文献

报道,对这些问题,医生能够直接回答的不到三分之一。这些问题涉及所有的临床医学专业,如治疗、危险因素和不良反应、诊断和预后,同时也与个体患者的具体情况高度相关。比如:

(1)运动疗法对膝关节炎的有效性和安全性如何?(不清楚是否有效或安全)

(2)抗生素治疗急性支气管炎有效吗?(有争议的话题)

(3)电动牙刷和手动牙刷,何者更有益于保持口腔健康?(有相互矛盾的答案)

如果你是一个临床医生,面对这些不清楚的,有争议的或答案相互矛盾的问题,你如何答复患者,如何找寻决策的支持?请各位思考,并和你的同桌讨论一下。

学生1:我也许会问问上级医生。

学生2:翻翻教科书。

学生3:上网找答案。

教师:还有吗?

学生4:和同事讨论。

教师:非常好!大家都有意识在给出草率的问题答案之前,尽量获得可靠的证据来支持我们的答案,无论这些支持是来源于上级医生、同事、教科书或是互联网。当然,不同的来源其可靠性和真实性可能是不同的,其后,我们将会详细讨论这些证据源和证据的可靠性和真实性。无论如何,我们这门课的关键内容就是"证据",所谓循证医学,就是基于证据的医学。以下是Sackett教授给出的定义。

(1)循证医学:指有意识地、明确地、审慎地利用现有最好的证据制定患者的诊治方案。实施循证医学意味着医生要参照最好的研究证据、临床经验和患者的意见。

(2)临床技能:指医生通过既往经验和临床实践所获得的对疾病的判断力和熟练的处理能力。高超的临床技能反映在许多方面,但特别反映在更高效正确的诊断以及在临床决策时对患者处境的周到考虑和对其病患的深切同情。

(3)可获得的最佳证据:指与临床相关的研究证据,这些证据可以来自基础医学研究,但更主要的是来自以患者为中心的临床研究。如关于诊断试验(包括临床检验)的准确性研究,预后标志物的把握度研究,治疗、康复和预防措施的有效性和安全性研究。来自临床研究的新证据不仅可以淘汰旧的、无效的诊断试验和治疗措施,而且还能以更准确、更有效和更安全的新措施取而代之。

（4）患者的价值观：指患者在其境遇下的个体的选择、关注点和期望,而这些在医生进行临床决策时应当被充分考虑和尊重。

6. 关于循证医学的讨论

互动 1.4：波浪和头脑风暴法

采用波浪技术将学生分组后,学生阅读指定的文献,小组讨论,完成小组任务,即用一张图来表现循证医学的优势与劣势。

教师：现在让我们放松一下,做一个波浪活动。请同学们从 1 到 5 依次报数（5 人/组,如果需要 4 人/组,则 1～4 报数,依此类推。假设全班有 50人）。记住自己的号码。

学生：（报数）

教师：很好,现在,所有报 1 的同学请起立,请坐下。所有报 2 的请起立,好,坐下。报 3 的同学起立,请坐。报 4 的同学请起立,请坐。报 5 的同学,请坐。非常好！现在我们请每一组同学依次起立、坐下,像波浪一样,每组同学起立时同时叫出自己的号码,并高举双臂,现在开始。

学生：（波浪）

教师：现在我们把报数相同的同学作为一个小组,每个小组找一张桌子围坐下,请阅读我分发的这篇文献,阅读完和小组成员讨论实践循证医学的优势和劣势分别是什么。

Sackett D L, et al. Evidence based medicine：what it is and what it isn't. BMJ, 1996, 3(12)：12.

学生：（阅读和讨论）

教师：（给每个小组发一张纸、一支笔和一份粘胶,每组笔的颜色不同。）请大家完成小组任务,画出如下图示,并将其贴在黑板上。每个小组推选一位代表,向全班解释你们的作品。

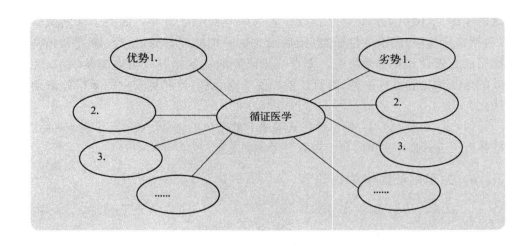

李红梅

Chapter 1

Introduction to EBM

Part I   Teaching Requirements

The first part of this session is an introduction to the course of EBM, including course outline, assessment, learning methods, and requirements for students as well. The second part is focused on EBM — a new clinic decision making model, and the three basic elements of EBM. By reading classical literatures and attaching to interactive activities, students could understand "what is EBM and what isn't, what are the advantages and disadvantages of practicing EBM".

1. Teaching aims

To discuss the concept of EBM, and its three elements. To investigate the necessity and feasibility, the advantages and disadvantages of practicing EBM.

2. Learning objectives

After completing this session, students should be able to:
(1) Define EBM.
(2) Describe the 3 elements of EBM.
(3) List the major advantages of practicing EBM.
(4) List the major disadvantages of practicing EBM.

3. Teaching methods

This session will use interactive teaching method, lecture and PPT presentation. Interactive techniques include marketing, background knowledge probe, think break, wave and brainstorming.

4. Reading materials

（1）Sackett D L，et al. Evidence based medicine：what it is and what it isn't. BMJ，1996，3（12）：12.

（2）Guyatt G，Rennie D. User's Guide to the Medical Literature：Essentials of Evidence-Based Clinical Practice. Chicago：AMA Pewaa，2001：3-22.

（3）Volk R J，Llewellyn-Thomas H，Stacey D，et al. Ten years of the International Patient Decision Aid Standards Collaboration：evolution of the core dimensions for assessing the quality of patient decision aids. Bmc Medical Informatics & Decision Making，2013，13 Suppl 2（S2）：S1.

Part Ⅱ　Teaching Design — 2 periods（80 minutes）

Teaching design of "Introduction to EBM"

No.	Content	Interactive technique/ teaching techniques	Descriptions	Time （minutes）
1	Introduction	Interaction 1.1：Marketing	Introduce teacher group to the class，ask students to introduce themselves to their deskmates，and ask some of them to introduce their deskmates to the class.	10
2	Survey before class	Interaction 1.2：Background knowledge probe	Distribute and collect "questionnaire before class" （see Appendix Ⅰ for questionnaire）.	10
3	Outline of the course and the course assessment	PPT presentation	Provide students with a brief outline of the course，as well as the assessment standards and requirements.	10
4	Introduce learning method	PPT presentation	Students make preparation before class and after class： 1. Emphasize the importance of reading articles prior to the class. Copies of the articles have been placed in the online class. （introduce how to log on the online class）.	10

（continued）

No.	Content	Interactive technique/ teaching techniques	Descriptions	Time (minutes)
			2. Emphasize to students on the importance of participating in interactions. 3. Introduce KWL chart to students. Ask them to complete it after class as a learning journal or diary). It will be talked over in pair and shared in the class in the next session (see Appendix II for KWL chart).	
5	Introduction to EBM	Interaction 1.3: Think break PPT slides	Introduce some clinical questions with no exact answers. Ask students to think about how to find the possible answers if they were a doctor. Then, elicit the concept of EBM.	20
6	Discussion on EBM	Interaction 1.4: Wave and brainstorming	Use "wave" to classify students into groups (5persons/group). Ask student to read the paper by Sackett D L individually for 5 minutes, then, students discuss "the advantages and disadvantages of practicing EBM" within the group, draw a mind map of the advantages and disadvantages.	20

Part III   Teaching Contents

1. Introduction

Introduce teacher group to the class, ask students to introduce themselves to their deskmates, and ask some of them to introduce their deskmates to the class.

Interaction 1.1 : Marketing

（This is the first class, through this interactive activity, the class would soon warm up, and students' ability of listening to others, remembering processing and reproducing information could be cultivated）

Teacher：You have known our team so far, now, I want you to talk with your deskmates for 3 minutes about your name, where you are from, your family and hobby, what you are good at, and others. Then I need some volunteers to sell their deskmates to the class.

… Time's up. Is there any volunteer who wants to introduce his or her deskmate to us? … Yes, please.

Student 1：This person next to me is a very cool guy who comes from Sri Lanka. He is the second child of the 5 children's family. He loves Chinese food very much, and likes to cook by himself.

Teacher：Do you ever taste his cooking? Yes? Taste good? Good! Anything else? No? Ok, next.

Student 2：My deskmate's name is Asha. She is from India, and she sings very well. I think she could be a super star if she didn't study medicine.

Teacher：Oh, really? can we ask this super star give us a short performance?

…

2. Questionnair survey before class

A questionnaire designed for this course is to investigate students' learning attitude and learning background. The questionnaire will be investigated before and after the course.（see Appendix I for questionnaire）.

Interaction 1.2 : Background knowledge probe

Teacher：Now I need two volunteers to help me distribute questionnaires.

This questionnaire helps understand your learning situation and needs, and it will not impact on your final scores, please fill in it truthfully. There are several options for each question, please tick the option which is fit for you, it can be multiselected if the choices are compatible.

Students: Should I write my name?

Teacher: No, you don't need to give your name. Please complete it in 10 mintues.

(Using questionnaire to acquire information is a good way to get feedback from students.)

3. Outline of the course

The course consists of 10 sessions, which provides an introduction to the key elements of EBM. They are:

(1) Introduction to Evidence-based Medicine.

(2) Asking an answerable question.

(3) Types of evidence (study) and grading of evidence.

(4) Searching for the medical evidence.

(5) Patients' value in clinical practice.

(6) Critical appraisal of therapeutic study.

(7) Critical appraisal of etiological study.

(8) Critical appraisal of diagnostic study.

(9) Critical appraisal of prognostic study.

(10) Introduction to systematic review and meta-analysis.

Performance of students consists of 3 aspects: students are expected to submit three assignments, each one being 15% of a total mark of 45%. Attendance ratio is worth 10%. The final test at the end of semester accounts for 45%.

4. Introduction to learning method

Student preparation before class and after class:

(1) Reading articles prior to the class. Copies of the articles have been placed in the online class. (Introduce how to log on the online class.)

(2) Participate actively in interactions.

(3) Complete KWL chart after everyday's learning (it will be the learning journal or diary). KWL chart will be talked over in pair and shared in the class in the next session (see Appendix II for KWL chart).

5. Introduction to EBM

Interaction 1.3 : Think break

Teacher: In real clinic situation, doctors always encounter lots of questions in their daily work, but they get answers for less than a third of them according to a document report. The questions are related to all medical specialties such as treatments, risk factors and side effects, diagnosis and prognosis and are highly specific to the individual patient's problem. Some clinical questions are as follows:

(1) Is exercise therapy effective and safe for knee osteoarthritis? (It is not clear.)

(2) Is it effective for antibiotics to treat acute bronchitis? (The answers always be controversial.)

(3) Powered toothbrushes vs. manual toothbrushes, which is more helpful for oral health? (May we find conflicting answers.)

If you are a clinician, how will you find the answer to these clinical questions without clear conclusions? Think about it and share your opinion with your deskmate.

Student 1: I will ask my superior doctor.

Student 2: Go and read the textbook.

Student 3: Quick glance at the Internet.

Teacher: Anything else?

Student 4: Discuss with my colleague.

Teacher: Very good! Everyone makes a conscious effort to get as much solid evidence as possible to back up our answers, whether it's from a superior doctor, a colleague, a textbook, or the Internet, before giving a hasty answer. Of course, the reliability and authenticity of different sources may vary, and we will discuss these sources and the reliability and authenticity of the evidence in detail later. Anyway, the key point of this course is about evidence. EBM is evidence-based medicine. Here is professor Sackett's definition.

(1) What is EBM? EBM has been described as "the conscientious,

explicit, judicious use of current best evidence in making decisions about the care of individual patients". The practice of evidence-based medicine integrates clinical expertise and patient values with the best available research evidence.

(2) Clinical expertise: "By individual clinical expertise we mean the proficiency and judgment that individual clinicians acquire through clinical experience and clinical practice. Increased expertise is reflected in many ways, but especially in more effective and efficient diagnosis and in the more thoughtful identification and compassionate use of individual patients predicaments rights, and preferences in making clinical decisions about their care. "

(3) Best available research evidence: By best available external clinical evidence we mean clinically relevant research, often from the basic sciences of medicine, but especially from patient-centered clinical research into the accuracy and precision of diagnostic tests (including the clinical examination), the power of prognostic markers, and the efficacy and safety of therapeutic, rehabilitative, and preventive regimens. External clinical evidence both invalidates previously accepted diagnostic tests and treatments and replaces them with new ones that are more powerful, more accurate, more efficacious, and safer.

Good doctors use both individual clinical expertise and the best available external evidence, and neither alone is enough.

(4) Patient values: This refers to the "unique preferences, concerns and expectations each patient brings to a clinical encounter and which must be integrated into clinical decisions if they are to serve the patient".

6. Discussion on EBM

Interaction 1.4 : Wave and brainstorming

After using wave technique to classify students into groups, students may read the assigned article, discuss within the group, then complete the group task: draw a mind map of advantages and disadvantages of EBM.

Teacher：Let do a wave activity. Now I need you to call a number from 1 to 5 one by one.(5 persons per group, if need 4 persons per group, call 1 to 4, and so on. The number of class students is assumed as 50) Please be sure to remember the number of yourself.

Students：(call number)

Teacher：Ok, all the students with number 1 stand up please, and sit down please. All number 2, stand up and sit down please. Number 3, and 4, and 5. Great! Now, I want the first number, that is, all students with number 1, of course, stand up and raise you arms and call out your number in the meantime, and sit down before the next number stand up. Number by number as one falls another rises.

Students：(do the wave)

Teacher：We have 5 groups now. The same number will be in the same group. Each group please find a table, and sit down, then read the following paper and discuss the advantages and disadvantages of practicing EBM.

Sackett D L, et al. Evidence based medicine: what it is and what it isn't. BMJ, 1996,3(12): 12.

Students：(read and discuss)

Teacher：(distribute papers, pens and stickers to groups, different group with different color) I need every group to draw a mind map like this and paste it on the blackboard. Every group should elect a representative to explain your map in front of class.

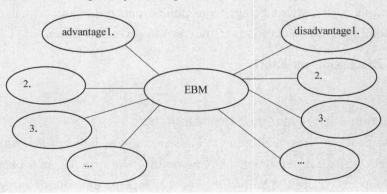

Li Hongmei

第 2 章

临床问题的提出

第一部分　教　学　要　求

此教学环节将介绍实践循证医学的步骤,以及"提出可回答的临床问题"的基本要素。

1. 教学目的

掌握根据临床情境提出可回答的临床问题的方法,以及一个好的临床问题的基本结构。

2. 学习目标

通过此环节的学习,学生能够:

(1) 描述实践循证医学的 5 个步骤。

(2) 理解一个好的临床问题的基本要素,即 PICO。

(3) 理解临床问题的类型。

(4) 能根据临床情境构建合适的可回答的临床问题。

3. 教学方法

此环节采用讲授法、PPT 演示和互动教学法,互动教学技术包括 TPS、概念匹配、一分钟作文和最糊涂的地方。

4. 阅读材料

Richardson W S，Wilson M C，Nishikawa J，et al. The well-built clinical question：a key to evidence-based decisions. Acp Journal Club，1995，123(3)：A12.

第二部分　教学设计——2 课时（80 分钟）

"临床问题的提出"教学设计表

序号	内　容	互动技术/教学技术	描　　　述	时间（分钟）
1	实践循证医学的 5 个步骤	PPT 演示	介绍实践循证医学的 5 个步骤	5
2	提出临床问题	互动 2.1：TPS	教师提供一个临床情境——Lisa，并提出问题，学生思考并与同桌讨论最佳答案，并向全班分享	20
3	一个好的临床问题的结构	PPT 演示	介绍一个好的临床问题的 4 个组成要素	10
4	临床问题的类型	PPT 演示	介绍与临床任务相关的常见临床问题的类型	10
5	"提问题"练习	互动 2.2：概念匹配	概念匹配能让学生更好地理解和掌握一个结构完好的临床问题的 4 个要素。提出好的临床问题是其后进行有效的证据检索的基础	25
6	复习	互动 2.3：一分钟作文和最糊涂的地方	学生花 1 分钟将"今天学习到的最重要的内容是什么"写在纸上，然后再花 1 分钟写下"今天学习到的内容中最让人困惑的是什么"。与同桌讨论，并与全班分享	10

第三部分　教　学　内　容

1. 实践循证医学的 5 个步骤

实践循证医学有以下 5 个步骤（5AS），本环节着重介绍第一步。

（1）提出可回答的临床问题。

（2）获得最佳临床证据。

（3）评价证据。

（4）应用证据于患者。

（5）EBM 实践后效评价。

2. 提出可回答的临床问题

互动 2.1：TPS

教师：我们来看一个临床情境：Lisa 是一个有活力的 77 岁的女性,几天前感到左膝关节疼痛。疼痛让她几乎不能行走。日前来到诊所看病。医生诊断为膝关节炎,并开了一些非甾体抗炎药给她。因为她曾有过消化性溃疡史,所以她询问医生是否可以不吃药,而是通过运动的方法进行治疗。医生比较怀疑运动疗法的效果,想知道有没有证据证实运动疗法对膝关节炎确实有效。

根据这个临床情境,思考医生面临决策,他遇到的问题是什么? 请各位在纸上写下医生会问的 3 个问题,并与你的同桌讨论哪一个问题比较好。

学生：(独立思考并与同伴讨论)

教师：时间到,有谁愿意与全班同学分享一下你们讨论的结果,请上台的同学把各自的问题写在黑板上。

学生 1：运动疗法对膝盖疼痛有好处吗?

学生 2：运动疗法对 77 岁的老年女性有用吗?

学生 3：对患膝关节炎的人来说,运动疗法是否能改善他们的情况?

教师：非常好! 好的问题是将来找寻答案进行临床决策的基础,我们一起来看一看这些问题提得好不好。

问题 1"运动疗法对膝盖疼痛有好处吗?"这个问题不够具体,我们不清楚患者的具体疾病是什么,"好处"的标准是什么。

问题 2"运动疗法有助于一个 77 岁的老年女性吗?"我们仍然不清楚这个患者的问题是什么,希望得到的治疗效果是什么?

问题 3"对患有膝关节炎人来说,运动疗法是否能改善他们的健康状况?"这个问题让我们知道了患者的疾病是什么,拟进行的干预措施是什么,但我们所期望达到的治疗效果是什么仍不清楚。期望的治疗效果可以是改善运动功能、缓解疼痛、提高舒适度,改善生存质量等。

所以,一个好的临床问题常常需要包含 4 个要素,即 PICO。

3. 构建良好的临床问题(PICO 问题)

一个构建良好的临床问题通常包括 4 个要素：① P,人群/患者/疾病;② I,干预/诊断试验/预后因素/暴露因素;③ C,比较;④ O,结局。

（1）人群/患者/疾病（P）

A．你将把查找到的信息用于何种患者？

B．你如何描述跟你目前患者相似的一组患者？

C．这组患者最重要的特征是什么？这些特征可能包括疾病的最初表现和并发症，有时也要涉及可能与诊断治疗有关的性别、年龄和种族等特征。

（2）干预/诊断试验/预后因素/暴露因素（I）

A．你考虑到的主要干预措施、诊断方法、预后因素或暴露因素是什么？

B．你将采取怎样的措施处理你的患者？开药？开诊断单？预约一个手术？

C．什么样的因素可能影响你的患者的预后？年龄？并发症？

D．你的患者曾经暴露在什么样的因素下？如是否吸烟等？

（3）比较（C）

A．与当前采取的干预措施相比，还有什么主要的替代方法？

B．你是否正在决定使用两种药中的哪一种？还是药物与非药物治疗、服药或不服药？抑或是两种诊断方法中的一种？

C．你的临床问题不必总是要有一个比较，有时也可以没有比较。

（4）结局（O）

A．你期望的结局是达到治疗目的、改善症状，还是有一定程度的影响？或诊断目的是什么？

B．你打算为患者做些什么？缓解或消除症状？减少不良反应事件？改善功能或测量指标？

构建良好的临床问题包括 4 个要素，并呈现以下结构：

患有（疾病）的人，与（比较）相比，采用（干预）可以提高/改善（结局）吗？

对于构建良好的临床问题我们还需要考虑问题的类型和研究类型。弄清楚这两点将有助于我们针对不同的问题类型，找寻最适合的临床证据。

4. 问题的类型和与之相应的临床研究任务（类型）

与临床研究任务有关的问题类型

研究类型	问　题　类　型
治疗研究	如何选择一种利大于弊的治疗
危害/病因研究	如何确定病因（包括医源性病因）
诊断研究	如果选择和解释诊断实验
预后研究	如何估计患者将来发展为各种不同后果或事件（痊愈、复发、恶化、伤残、并发症和死亡等）的概率

5. "提问题"练习

互动 2.2：概念匹配

教师在即时贴上写好一些关键词,学生将其组织成为一个有意义的结构

教师: 大家还记得 Lisa 吗? 还记得你们曾经问过的三个问题吗? 它们是好的临床问题吗? 你们忽略了哪些重要的要素?

让我们一起来基于 Lisa 的情况再构建一次临床问题,记得用 PICO 结构,考虑下列问题,并完成填空:

(1) 这个问题的主要组成要素是什么?

(2) 这是一个什么类型的临床问题,即是关于治疗、病因、预后还是诊断的问题? 不同的临床问题将寻求最好的研究设计来回答,下周我们将关注于此。

对患有(疾病)的人,与(比较)相比,采用(干预)是否能改善(结局)?

有谁愿意来完成这个填空的任务?

学生: 对患有(膝关节炎)的人,与(药物疗法或非甾体抗炎药)相比,采用(运动疗法)是否能(提高患者的舒适度和运动能力)?

教师: 棒极了! 你能告诉我们这个问题的类型是什么吗? 是治疗性问题、病因、诊断,还是预后问题?

学生: 治疗性问题。

教师: 正确! 现在,我手里有一些即时贴,每张上面都写着一些术语,一些是疾病的名称或人群的名称,一些是干预的措施或药物的名称,一些是暴露因素或结局,还有一些是问题的类型。你们每人上来拿一张,然后互相寻找自己的同伴,直到形成一个完整的临床问题,即包含四个要素及问题的类型。找到小组成员的同学将你们小组的字条按 PICO＋问题类型的顺序贴在黑板上,我们看看哪一个小组最快。最后我们再请每个小组的 P 作为代表将你们的问题念给全班同学听。(字条如下:)

吸烟	不吸烟	肺癌	发病率	病因问题
成年人	电动牙刷	手动牙刷	口腔健康	预后问题
急性支气管炎	抗生素	抗病毒制剂	有效性和安全性	治疗问题
老年膝关节炎患者	抗炎药 A	抗炎药 B	胃肠道的副作用	

6. 复习：用 KWL 表完成一分钟作文

学生用 10 分钟的时间回顾所学的内容,完成 KWL 表,与同伴讨论并分享。

互动 2.3：一分钟作文和最糊涂的地方

一分钟作文:学生花 1 分钟写下一个具体的问题,一般如"今天学习到的最重要的内容是……"

最糊涂的地方:与上面提到的 1 分钟写作相似,只是写作内容变为"今天最让我困惑的是……"二者都适合用于课堂结束前的复习。

教师: 现在我们要花 10 分钟复习一下今天所学的内容。首先给各位 5 分钟的时间完成你们的 KWL 表,然后我要向你们提问。

学生: (完成 KWL 表)

教师: 好,现在请各位用 1 分钟的时间把今天学到的、你认为最重要的内容写在纸上,然后与你的同桌分享和讨论。

时间到,有谁能告诉我们你的同桌认为最重要的内容是什么?

学生 1: 我同桌认为她今天学到的最重要的内容是一个好的临床问题的结构。

教师: 很好!现在,再请各位花 1 分钟把你认为今天最让你困惑的内容写下来,并与同桌分享和讨论。

时间到,有谁愿意告诉我们自己同桌写的是什么?

学生 2: 我的同桌认为最困惑他的是:我们提出一个临床问题的时候,为什么还要弄清楚这个问题的类型。

教师: 非常好!有谁能够帮这个同学解答一下疑问呢?

学生 3: 弄清楚问题的类型有助于针对问题寻找答案……

教师: 以及确定可以回答这个问题的临床证据的类型。其后的教学中我们将详细解答这个内容。

好,下课时间到了,下周见!

李红梅　李　咏

Chapter 2

Asking an Answerable Clinical Question

Part I Teaching Requirements

This session will introduce the steps of practicing EBM, and the principle of "asking an answerable clinical question".

1. Teaching aims

To understand the principle of "ask an answerable question" for a clinical scenario and the structure of a good clinical question.

2. Learning objectives

After completing this session, students should be able to:

(1) Discribe the 5 steps of practicing EBM.

(2) Understand the components of a good answerable question (PICO).

(3) Understand the types of questions.

(4) Construct appropriate answerable questions according to the clinical scenarios.

3. Teaching methods

This session will use PPT presentation, lecture and interactive teaching method. Interactive teaching techniques include TPS, concept matching, one-minute paper and muddiest point.

4. Reading materials

Richardson W S, Wilson M C, Nishikawa J, et al. The well-built clinical question: a key to evidence-based decisions. Acp Journal Club, 1995, 123(3): A12.

Part II　Teaching Design — 2 periods（80 minutes）

Teaching design of "Asking an Answerable Question"

No.	Content	Interactive technique/ teaching techniques	Descriptions	Time （minutes）
1	5 steps of practicing EBM	PPT presentation	Introduction to the 5 steps of practicing EBM.	5
2	Ask clinical questions	Interaction 2.1：TPS	Provide a clinical scenario： Lisa. Teacher asks questions. Students share and compare possible answers to a question with a partner before addressing the class.	20
3	Structure of a good answerable clinical question	PPT presentation	Introduction to the four components of a good answerable clinical question.	10
4	Introduction to the type of clinical question	PPT presentation	Introduction to the most common types of questions related to clinical tasks.	10
5	"Asking question" practicing	Interaction 2.2：Concept matching	Concept matching allows students to better understand the 4 components of a well-built clinical question， which is the basic step of conducting a good evidence retrieval.	25
6	Review	Interaction 2.3：One-minute paper and muddiest point	Students write for one minute on "what was the most important thing you learned today?" Then， take another minute to write "what is the most confusing thing you learned today?" Discuss in pair and share in class.	10

Part III　Teaching Contents

1. 5 steps of practicing EBM

The practice of EBM requires the following 5 steps（5AS）. This session will focus on the first step.

(1) Asking an answerable clinical question.

(2) Acquiring the best evidence.

(3) Appraising the evidence.

(4) Applying the evidence to the patient.

(5) Assessing the after-effect of EBM practice.

2. Ask clinical questions

Interaction 2.1 : TPS

Teacher: Let's look at this clinical scenario: Lisa is a vigorous 77 year old female. Several days ago, she developed pain in her left knee, making it hard for her to walk. She came to the clinic. The doctor made the diagnosis of osteoarthritis and gave her prescription of non-steroidal anti-inflammatory drugs. Because of her digestive ulcer history, she asked if she could begin a course of physical therapy instead of taking medicine.

The doctor is suspicious of this suggestion. He wants to know whether there is any proof that physical therapy does her any good to this problem.

What is the question according to this scenario? Please think of it and list at least 3 questions you want to ask. Then, discuss with your partner about which the best clinical question is.

Students: (think independently and discuss in pair)

Teacher: Time's up. Is there any volunteer to share your questions in front of class? Please write down your questions on the blackboard.

Student 1: Is exercise therapy good for a painful knee?

Student 2: Can physical therapy help an elderly 77-year-old female?

Student 3: For people with osteoarthritis, can physical therapy improve their health conditions?

Teacher: Good job! A good question is the basis of looking for the answer, and making a good clinic decision. Let's look at the questions.

Q1"Is physical therapy good for a painful knee? "This question is not specific enough. We still want to know the patient's problem. Also, what are the criteria for "good"?

Q2"Can physical therapy help an elderly 77-year-old female?"We still want to know what the patient's problem is. What is the expected outcome?

Q3"For people with osteoarthritis, can physical therapy improve their health conditions?"We know the patient's problem, the intervention, but the expected outcome is still not so clear. Expected therapeutic effects include improved exercise performance, pain relief, enhanced comfort, and improved quality of life.

Therefore, a good clinical problem often needs to contain four elements, namely, PICO.

3. Structure of a good clinical question (PICO question)

A well-built question usually contains 4 components: ① P, population/patient/problem; ② I, intervention/diagnostic test/prognostic factor/exposure; ③ C, comparison; ④ O, outcomes.

（1）Population/patient/problem（P）

A. What is the group of patients that you will apply the information to?

B. How would you describe a group of patients similar to yours?

C. What are the most important characteristics of the patients? This may include the primary problem disease, or co-existing conditions. Sometimes the sex, age or race of a patient might be relevant to the diagnosis or treatment of a disease.

（2）Intervention/diagnostic test/prognostic factor/exposure（I）

A. Which main intervention, diagnostic test, prognostic factor, or exposure is you consideration?

B. What do you want to do to the patient? A prescription? Make a diagnosis? Book an operation?

C. What factors may influence the prognosis of the patient? Age? Co-existing problems?

D. What was the patient exposed to? Is he (she) a cigarette smoker?

（3）Comparison（C）

A. What are the main options to compare with the intervention?

B. Are you deciding to give one of the two drugs? Pharmacotherapy vesus non-pharmaceutical therapy, taking or not taking medication, or choosing one of the two diagnostic methods?

C. Your clinical question does not always have to have a specific comparison.

（4）Outcomes（O）

A. What can you hope to accomplish, improve or affect, or what is your purpose of diagnosis?

B. What are you trying to do for the patient? Relieve or eliminate the symptoms? Reduce the number of adverse events? Improve function or test scores?

A well-built clinical question has these 4 components which formulate an answerable question from them. The structure of the question might look like this:

For people with （disease）does （intervention）affect （outcome） compared to （comparison, if any）?

In addition, for a "well-built clinical question", we also need to consider the type of question and the type of study. These information can be helpful in focusing on the question and determining the most appropriate type of clinical evidence.

4. Types of questions related to clinical tasks

The most common types of questions related to clinical tasks

Type of study	Type of question
Therapy study	How to select treatments offered to patients that do more good than harm
Harm/etiology study	How to identify the cause for disease （including iatrogenic forms）
Diagnosis study	How to select and interpret diagnostic tests
Prognosis study	How to estimate the probability that the patient will develop into various consequences or events （recovery, recurrence, deterioration, disability, complications, death, etc.）

5. "Asking question"practicing

Interaction 2.2： Concept matching

Teacher writes keywords on the sticky notes and then students organize them into a meaningful structure.

Teacher：Do you remember Lisa? Remember those three questions you asked，are they good clinical questions? which component you have missed?

Let's formulate an answerable question based on Lisa again（use PICO structure），thinking of the following questions and filling in the blanks：

（1）What are the main components of the question?

（2）What type of question is it，i.e. a question about treatment，etiology，prognosis or diagnosis? The best study design in order to answer the type of question will be given. And next week we will focus on this.

For people with（disease）does（intervention）affect（outcome）compared to（comparison，if any）?

Anyone who wants to be the volunteer to complete this task?

Student：For patients with disease（knee osteoarthritis）does（physical therapy）affect（comfort and mobility）compared to（drug therapy or non-steroidal anti-inflammatory drugs）?

Teacher：Brilliant! Could you please tell me what type of question it is? Is it a therapy，etiology，diagnosis or prognosis question?

Student：Therapy question.

Teacher：Right! Now，here are some sticky notes on which I have written different terms. Some of them are diseases or population，some of them are interventions or drugs，exposures or outcomes and some of them are question types. Each of you come and pick up one note. Then you can go around and find your partners，finally，form a completed well-built clinical question，which contains 4 components and question type. Students who have found the members of your group，please stick your notes by the order of PICO+question type on the blackboard. Let's see which group is the fastest one. Finally, we will ask P of every group to be the representative to read the whole question in public group by group. (The cards will be as follows.)

Smoking	Non-smoking	lung cancer	Incidence rate	Etiology question
Adults	Powered toothbrushes	Manual toothbrushes	Oral health	Prognosis question
Acute bronchitis	Antibiotics	Antiviral agents	Effectiveness and safety	Therapy question
Elderly patients with OA knee		One NSAID	Another NSAID	GIT side effects

6. Review: one-minute paper with KWL chart

Students spend 10 minutes going over the lessons, completing KWL chart, discussing and sharing it.

Interaction 2.3 : One-minute paper and muddiest point

One-minute paper: Students write for 1 minute on a specific question, which might be generalized to "what was the most important thing you learned today".

Muddiest point: Like the minute paper, however, use the "most confusing thing" instead. Both are best used at the end of the class session.

Teacher: Now, we will spend the last 10 minutes to go over the lessons, please complete your KWL chart at first, you have 5 minutes. Then I will ask you some questions.

Students: (completing KWL chart)

Teacher: Now, I need you to write for one minute on what was the most important thing you learned today and talk to your deskmates.

Time's up. Is there anyone who wants to tell us what the most important thing your deskmate learned?

Student 1：My deskmate thinks the most important thing she learned is the structure of a well-built clinical question.

Teacher：Good! Now I need you to write for one minute on what is the most confusing thing you learned today and talk to your deskmates.

Time is up. Is there anyone who want to tell us what is the most confusing thing your deskmate learned?

Student 2：My deskmate thinks the most confusing thing is why we also need to define the question type when we build a clinical question.

Teacher：Great! May I ask someone to explain this for her?

Student 3：To know the type of question can be helpful in focusing on the question …

Teacher：And determining the most appropriate type of clinical evidence，we will explain it in detail later on.

Ok，it's time to say goodbye. See you next week!

Li Hongmei   Li Yong

第 3 章

证据类型和分级

第一部分　教　学　要　求

本教学环节首先介绍了临床研究设计,包括研究设计的类型以及他们的优缺点。其次,由研究设计的优缺点推演了证据的级别并引出了证据金字塔。最后,通过实例让学生将证据级别的思想运用到具体的循证医学实践中。

1. 教学目的

明确循证医学证据的类型(基于研究设计)以及证据的级别。

2. 学习目标

通过此环节的学习,学生能够:

(1) 列出研究设计,包括不同研究设计的类型和各自的优劣势。

(2) 列出证据的类型。

(3) 描述证据的分级。

3. 教学方法

此环节采用讲授法、PPT 演示和互动教学法,互动教学技术包括 TPS、挑选胜利者。

4. 阅读材料

Murad M H,Asi N,Alsawas M,et al. New evidence pyramid. Evidence-based Medicine,2016,21(4):125-127.

第二部分   教学设计——2 课时（80 分钟）

"证据类型和分级"教学设计表

序号	内　容	互动技术/教学技术	描　　　　　述	时间（分钟）
1	案例	互动 3.1：TPS	介绍具体临床案例后，采用 TPS 互动技术，让学生思考并设计一个临床实验来研究案例中遇到的问题，然后配对讨论，最后请几名学生在全班分享成果	15
2	临床研究设计简介	PPT 演示	介绍临床研究的设计类型	20
3	关于临床研究设计的讨论	互动 3.2：TPS	让学生思考并两两讨论：以上研究设计中，哪种研究设计得到的结果更真实可靠及其原因。然后请 1～2 名学生向全班分享他们的观点	15
4	各临床研究设计的优缺点	PPT 演示	总结各临床研究设计的优缺点	10
5	证据金字塔介绍	PPT 演示	通过 PPT，由以上讨论的各研究设计优缺点推演出证据的级别并引出证据金字塔	5
6	实践	互动 3.3：挑选胜利者	将全班分成若干小组，每个小组就课程开始时的临床案例构建循证医学的问题，然后根据课堂上给出的检索结果讨论怎样对其进行初筛，将他们的答案写在纸上。然后每个组交换至相邻的组并评价相邻组的答案。允许他们进行观点整合并选出最佳答案向全班展示	15

第三部分   教 学 内 容

1. 临床案例

Jack，35 岁，咳嗽、咯痰 2 天。既往史无特殊。他到医院寻求帮助。通过检查,你的初步诊断为急性支气管炎。现在他的实验室检查结果还未出来,你想要知道这种情况下使用抗生素是否有益?

互动 3.1: TPS

　　教师: 你将怎样回答这个问题? 当然,你可以在文献中找到他人研究提供的证据,或者,你也可以自己做一个实验来找到答案。

　　现在,假设大家都是致力于研究急性支气管炎患者使用抗生素是否有益的研究者。现在有 100 位患者作为研究对象,请同学们思考怎样设计自己的研究、应该注意哪些方面,并和同桌进行讨论。最后由几位同学在全班分享他们的方案。

　　学生组 1: 我们的设计是让所有患者服用抗生素,观察数天后他们是否治愈。

　　教师: 很好,但是有一个问题就是你怎样确定这些患者是被药物"治愈"的而不是"自愈"的呢?

　　学生组 1: 可能确定不了。

　　教师: 对的,因为我们没有对照组进行比较。还有其他想法吗?

　　学生组 2: 我和同桌讨论后认为我们应该将 100 位患者分成 2 组,1 组服用抗生素,1 组不服用,观察数天后他们的结局。

　　教师: 很好,那如何将患者进行分组呢? 按照你自己的意愿? 还是其他方法? 非常好,随机分配。

　　(通过这种方法,促使学生们深刻思考研究设计,并引起他们对下面内容的兴趣。)

2. 临床研究设计简介

　　临床研究有两大领域:实验性研究和观察性研究。根据是由研究者来分配暴露因素(如治疗)还是研究者仅对临床实践进行了观察,就能迅速分辨研究所属的领域。前者为实验性研究,如随机对照实验,后者为观察性研究。对于观察性研究来说,如果有比较或者说对照组,就称为分析性研究,如病例对照研究和队列研究;如果没有对照组,则称为描述性研究,如病例报告、病例系列报告和横断面调查。

　　(1)描述性研究:处于研究的最下端,常常是开启一个新的医学研究领域的开端。研究者用其描述疾病的发病率(Ir)、患病率(Pr)、自然病程和可能的决定因素，描述疾病和患者的特征，并产生关于疾病的假设。常见的描述性研究包括病例报告、病例系列报告、横断面调查等。

（2）分析性研究

A. 病例对照研究：

- 选择一组患有所研究疾病的人作为病例组，一组未患有该疾病的人作为对照组，两组特征基本一致。
- 比较两组间既往暴露的差异。

B. 队列研究：

- 队列是可以区分亚群特征的人群。
- 研究者对两组随访适当长的时间。
- 在研究之初，一组暴露于某一特定因素或接受某一特定治疗，一组没有。
- 经过适当长时间的随访，比较两组之间所研究疾病的发病率或死亡率差异。

（3）实验性研究：随机对照试验（RCT）。

- 确定适用于本问题的研究对象。
- 将研究对象分成两组或多组。
- 对照组可以给予目前公认的最佳干预措施。
- 在理想状态下，试验组和对照组的研究对象的特征应有同质性，尤其是那些可能影响疾病结局的特征。
- 为了达到上述的同质性，研究对象应该是随机分配到各组中的。

3. 关于临床研究设计的讨论

互动 3.2：TPS

教师： 请同学们思考以上研究设计中哪种研究设计得到的结果更真实可靠，分析原因及它们可以用在什么情况下。然后同学们两两讨论，最后我们请 1 位同学在全班进行分享。

学生： 我认为 RCT 提供的结果更真实，利用随机对照试验我们可以将患者随机进行分组，这就保证了每组间的特征基本相似。

教师： 很好，实际上 RCT 还有很多其他的优点，同时它也有缺点。因此并不是所有情况下我们都可以运用 RCT 这种研究设计。现在我们来讨论各个常见研究类型的优缺点。

（通过 TPS 这种方式，教师能引导学生进一步思考各种研究设计的优缺点，让他们能对下面的内容产生兴趣。）

4. 各研究设计的优缺点

（1）个案报道

A. 对单个病例症状、体征、诊断、治疗和随访的仔细而详细的报告。

B. 为发现新病种和副作用提供线索（例如，个案报道为口服避孕药增加静脉血栓栓塞风险提供线索）。

（2）病例系列报告

A. 病例系列（也称临床系列）是一种跟踪已知暴露的患者，如接受过相似治疗或检查其医疗记录以了解暴露和结局的描述性研究。

B. 是对病案的有效记录。

C. 通过对系列病例的分析来认识疾病。

D. 通常用于研究疾病的症状体征、定义疾病、临床教学等。

（3）病例对照研究

A. 优点：① 物力耗费少，出结果快；② 往往是罕见疾病病因研究的唯一设计模型。

B. 缺点：① 依赖于回忆或记录来确定暴露；② 容易受回忆偏倚、选择偏倚影响。

（4）队列研究

A. 优点：① 符合伦理；② 可以确定事件的时间和方向性；③ 与 RCT 相比，更容易执行、花费金钱更少。

B. 缺点：① 容易引入混杂因素；② 盲法较难实现；③ 无法进行随机化分配。

（5）随机对照试验

A. 优点：① 前瞻性的对照；② 控制偏倚；③ 诊断和实施标准化；④ 可比性好。

B. 缺点：① 样本量大；② 随访时间长（可能有失访）；③ 时间成本、经济成本高；④ 可能存在的伦理学问题。

（6）系统评价：也叫系统文献综述或结构式文献综述（SLR），是针对某一具体的问题，系统全面地识别、筛选和严格评价相关研究，并对原始研究的数据进行收集、分析和整合，最终形成的综述性文献。对高质量的随机对照试验的系统评价在循证医学中非常重要。

5. 证据金字塔

证据的分级有许多标准，其中 2001 年美国纽约州立大学下属医学中心推出的证据金字塔，将证据分为 9 个级别，初学者较容易把握，是证据检索和评价的便捷工具。

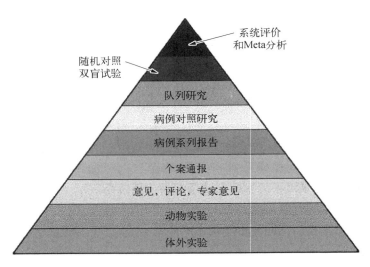

证据金字塔

6. 实践

在学习了有关常用的研究设计及其优缺点、证据金字塔等内容后,学生们应该能够利用这些知识解决在实践循证医学时遇到的问题。

互动3.3： 挑选胜利者

将学生们进行分组,每个组根据我们这节课开始时的案例构建出一个循证医学的问题,然后根据以下检索结果讨论怎样对其进行初筛,并将答案写在纸上。然后每个组交换至相邻的组并评价相邻组的答案。允许他们进行观点整合并选出最佳答案向全班展示。

教师:现在请同学们按从1到10进行报数(这里我们将学生分为10个组,如果要分为8个组则从1到8进行报数,以此类推,假设全班有50名学生)。请同学们记住自己的报数。

学生:(报数)

教师:现在,所有报数1的同学为一组,所有报数2的同学为一组,所有报数3的同学为一组……

每个组的同学,请再次思考本节课开始的案例,利用之前学习过的PICO构建一个循证医学的问题,并写出如果我们的检索结果如下图,怎样对结果进行初筛。将你们的答案写在纸上。

(数分钟后)

教师：现在请每个组交换至相邻的组并评价相邻组的答案，将你们自己的答案留在桌上。大家可以和其他组的答案进行观点整合并选出最佳答案向全班展示。

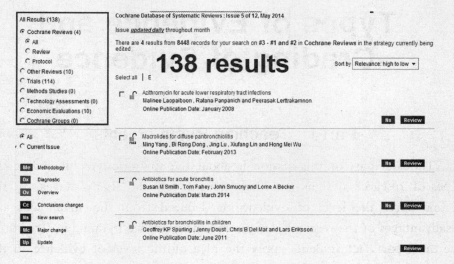

检索结果

（数分钟后）

教师：现在我们需要每组同学派一位代表来展示各组的答案，然后我们大家选出最佳的一个作为优胜者。

学生：（演示）

优 胜 答 案

P（患者）	I（干预措施）	C（对照）	O（结局）
患急性支气管炎的成人	抗生素	安慰剂/空白对照	疗效和安全性

根据证据金字塔，系统评价位于证据级别顶端，因此我们应该先浏览系统评价。

教师：非常好，我们可以先浏览系统评价，这里的 Cochrane Review 和 Other Review 都属于系统评价，所以我们可以先浏览这些结果，总共是 14 条记录。

（让学生分组对刚刚学习的知识进行讨论并评价其他学生的答案是一个帮助学生们理解知识点的很好的方法。）

谭睿璟

Chapter 3

Types of Evidence and Grading of Evidence

Part I   Teaching Requirements

The first part of this session is about the study designs, including the types of research designs and their advantages and disadvantages. In the second part, the level of evidence is deduced from the advantages and disadvantages of the research designs and the Evidence Pyramid is derived. In the third part, let students apply the idea of the level of evidence to the practice of EBM.

1. Teaching aims

To crystallize the types of evidence based on study design and the grading of evidence.

2. Learning objectives

After completing this session, students should be able to:

(1) List the research designs, including the types of research designs and their advantages and disadvantages.

(2) List types of evidence.

(3) Describe the grading of evidence.

3. Teaching methods

This session will use lecture, PPT presentation and interactive teaching method. Interactive teaching techniques include TPS and pick the winner.

4. Reading materials

Murad M H, Asi N, Alsawas M, et al. New evidence pyramid. Evidence-based Medicine, 2016, 21(4): 125 – 127.

Part II   Teaching Design — 2 periods (80 minutes)

Teaching design of "Types of Evidence and Grading of Evidence"

No.	Content	Interactive techniques/ teaching techniques	Descriptions	Time (minutes)
1	Scenario	Interaction 3.1: TPS	After the introduction to specific clinical cases, TPS interactive technology is used to ask students to think and design a clinical experiment to study the problems existing in the cases, and then discuss in pairs. Finally, several students are invited to share the results in the class.	15
2	Introduction to clinical study designs	PPT presentation	Introduce clinical study designs to students.	20
3	Discussion on study designs	Interaction 3.2: TPS	Ask students to think and discuss in pairs " which study design can provide the most valid result, tell the reason". Then ask one or two students to share their ideas in front of the class.	15
4	Advantages and disadvantages of each study design	PPT presentation	Summarize the advantages and disadvantages of each study design.	10
5	Introduction to the evidence pyramid	PPT presentation	Through the PPT, the advantages and disadvantages of each research design discussed above are used to deduce the grade of evidence and lead to the Evidence Pyramid.	5

(**continued**)

No.	Content	Interactive techniques/ teaching techniques	Descriptions	Time （minutes）
6	Practicing	Interaction 3.3: Pick the winner	Divide the class into groups and ask all groups to build a formulated question and find out how to screen primarily the evidence according to the scenario which has been given, and write their answers on papers. Each group was then swapped to an adjacent group and evaluated for answers from the adjacent group. Allow them to integrate their ideas and choose the best answer to present to the class.	15

Part III   Teaching Contents

1. A scenario

Jack is a 35 year-old adult whose medical history was unremarkable. He has been coughing with sputum for two days. He comes to the clinic asking for help. You give him a diagnosis of acute bronchitis. Now the results of his laboratory examinations are not available yet, so you want to know whether antibiotics are beneficial or not?

Interaction 3.1: TPS

Teacher: What will you do to answer this question? Yeah, you may find out evidence in literature which is the research results of others or you may also do a research by yourself to find out the answers.

Now, suppose you were researchers, who want to find out whether antibiotic is good or not for patients with acute bronchitis. There are 100 patients you could observe. Please think about how to regulate the study and what are the tips you would give attention to while regulating the study, and then talk to your partner about your idea, after that, we will ask someone to share his idea or his partner's in front of the class.

Student 1: We will ask them to take antibiotics and to see if they would be cured after several days.

Teacher: Good, but there is a question. If the patients were "cured", would you be sure that they were cured by the drugs or healed by themselves?

Student 1: Maybe not.

Teacher: Good, because there is no comparison. Anyone else?

Student 2: After the discussing, my partner and I both think we would divide these 100 patients into two groups, one group takes antibiotics and the other does not, and to see their outcomes in several days.

Teacher: Very good, and how will you divide your patients into groups? Depend on your thought? Or else? Very good, randomly.

(Through this way, students can think about the study design deeply, and they would be interested in the following content.)

2. Introduction to clinical study designs

There are two major categories in clinical study, experimental research and observational research. The category of a study can be quickly identified depending on whether the researcher allocates exposure factors (e. g., treatment) or whether the researcher merely conducts observation. The former is experimental research, such as randomized controlled trail, and the latter is observational research. For observational research, if there is a comparison, or a control group, it is called analytical research, such as case-control study and cohort study. If there is no control group, it is called descriptive research, such as case report, case series, and cross-sectional survey.

(1) Descriptive research: Descriptive research is at the bottom of the research scale. It is often the first research to be undertaken when we enter a new field of medicine. Researchers use it to describe the incidence rate (Ir), prevalence rate (Pr), natural course of disease, and possible determinants, to

describe the characteristics of the disease and the patient, and to generate hypotheses about the disease. Common descriptive research includes case report, case series, cross-sectional survey, etc.

(2) Analytical research

A. Case control study:

● A group of people with a disease under investigation was selected as the case group, and another group without the disease as the control group. The characteristics of the two groups are basically the same.

● Compare the past exposures of both groups.

B. Cohort study:

● Cohorts are defined populations that, as a whole, are followed in an attempt to determine distinguishing subgroup characteristics.

● Researchers identify and compare two groups over a period of time.

● At the start of the study, one of the groups is exposed to a particular factor or receives a particular treatment, and the other does not.

● At the end of a certain amount of time, the differences in morbidity or mortality between the two groups are compared by researchers.

(3) Experimental research: randomized controlled trail (RCT).

● Define a study population suitable for answering the question.

● Divide the study population into two or more groups.

● The control group may be offered the best known alternative.

● In the ideal trial, the study and control populations are similar, especially in characteristics impacting on disease outcomes.

● To achieve this similarity, individuals in the study are assigned randomly to the groups.

3. Discussion on clinical study designs

Interaction 3.2 : TPS

Teacher: Now please think about which of the research design can provide the most valid result, and why. To what circumstances are they available? Then share your ideas with your partners before sharing them in front of the class.

Student: I think RCT could provide us with the most valid result, because we may divide our objectives into groups randomly. This may make sure that the characters of each group are similar.

Teacher: Very good, and there are many advantages of RCT. However, there are also disadvantages. So RCT is not always available. Now let's discuss the advantages and disadvantages of each.

(Through this way, the teacher can lead the students to think about the advantages and disadvantages of each study design deeply, and they would develope interest in the following content.)

4. Advantages and disadvantages of each

(1) Case report

A. Careful and detailed report of the symptoms, signs, diagnosis, treatment, and follow-up of the profile of a single patient.

B. Can provide clues in the identification of a new disease or adverse effects of exposures [i.e. a case report gives the clue that oral contraceptive (OC) use increases the risk of venous thromboembolism].

(2) Case series

A. A case series (also known as a clinical series) is a descriptive research that tracks patients with known exposure, such as patients who were given a similar treatment, or examines their medical records for exposure and outcome.

B. A case-series is, effectively, a register of cases.

C. Analyse cases together to learn about the disease.

D. Series are of value in epidemiology for studying symptoms and signs, creating case definitions, clinical education.

(3) Case control study

A. Advantages: ① quick and cheap; ② the only feasible method for very rare disorders or those with long lag between exposure and outcome.

B. Disadvantages: ① reliance on recall or records to determine exposure status; ② potential bias: recall, selection.

(4) Cohort study

A. Advantages: ① ethically safe; ② can establish timing and directionality of events；③ administratively easier and cheaper than RCT.

B. Disadvantages：① exposure may be linked to a hidden confounder；② blinding is difficult；③ randomization not present.

（5）RCT

A. Advantages：① a prospective controlled design；② controlling bias；③ standardized process of diagnosis and implementation；④ high comparability.

B. Disadvantages：① large trials；② long term follow-up（possible losses）；③ expensive：time and money；④ possible ethical questions.

（6）Systematic review：also systematic literature review or structured literature review（SLR）. A review of the literature，in which there is a clearly formulated question，and systematic and explicit methods are used to identify，select and critically appraise relevant research，and to collect，analyze and synthesize data from the orginal studies that are included in the review. Systematic reviews of high-quality randomized controlled trials are crucial to EBM.

5. The Evidence Pyramid

There are many criteria for the levels of evidence. Among those，the Evidence Pyramid raised by SUNY Downstate Medial Center devides evidence into nine levels. It is much easier for beginners to understand，so it becomes a convenient tool to acquire and appraise evidence.

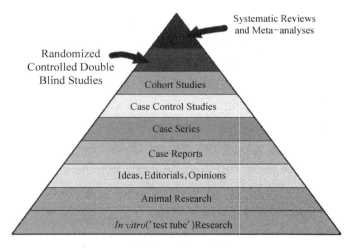

Evidence Pyramid

6. Practice

After learning some commonly-used study designs, their advantages and disadvantages, and the Evidence Pyramid, students should be able to use them when practicing EBM.

Interaction 3.3 : Pick the winner

Classify students into groups. Ask each group to build a formulated question and find out how to screen primarily the evidence according to the scenario which has been given, to write their answers on paper. Each group is then swapped to an adjacent group and evaluates the answers from the adjacent group. Allow them to integrate their ideas and choose the best answer to present to the class.

Teacher: Now I need you to call out the number from 1 to 10 one by one. (Here we divide students into 10 groups, if needed, 8 groups, call out from 1 to 8, and so on, the number of the students in the class is assumed as 50) Please be sure to remember the number of yourself.

Students: (call out the number)

Teacher: Now, all number 1 students get together to be a group, all number 2s a group, all number 3s a group ...

All the groups, please go through the scenario given at the beginning of this class, and ask a formulated question with PICO format first and tell how to screen primarily the evidence if the search result is as follows. Write down your answers on the paper.

(after several minutes)

Teacher: Now, please switch to an adjacent group and evaluate their answers. Leave your answers on the table. You can integrate their ideas or select the best answer as yours.

(after several minutes)

Teacher: Now we need one student to be on behalf of his/her group to demonstrate their answer. And we will pick out the best one as the winner.

Students: (demonstrating)

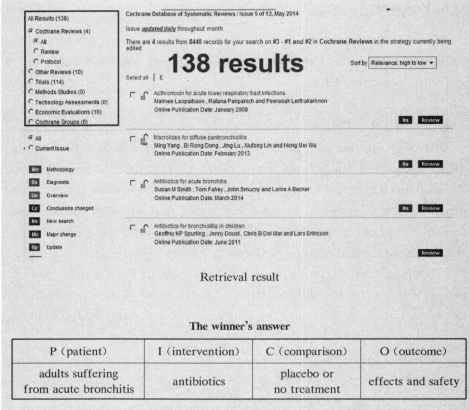

Retrieval result

The winner's answer

P (patient)	I (intervention)	C (comparison)	O (outcome)
adults suffering from acute bronchitis	antibiotics	placebo or no treatment	effects and safety

According to the Evidence Pyramid，systematic review is on the top of Evidence Pyramid，so we can go through systematic review first.

Teacher：Excellent，we can go through systematic review first，and here，Cochrane review and other review are both systematic review，so we can have a look at them first. Here are 14 results.

（Having students discuss what they have just learned in groups and evaluate the answers of other students is a good way to help students understand the knowledge points.）

Tan Ruijing

第 4 章

医学证据检索

第一部分　教　学　要　求

本教学环节主要是关于证据检索的步骤,包括每个步骤的讨论、常用数据库的使用介绍及检索的实践。

1. 教学目的

学习和实践获取循证医学证据的基本步骤及常用循证医学资源的使用。

2. 学习目标

通过此环节的学习,学生能够:

（1）理解证据资源的 6S 模型。

（2）运用检索证据的基本步骤。

（3）能够通过常用循证医学资源如 Cochrane Library 和 PubMed Clinical Queries 检索到证据。

3. 教学方法

此环节采用讲授法、PPT 演示及互动教学法,互动教学技术包括创造性会话、拼字、头脑风暴、利弊面和传递问题。

4. 阅读材料

（1）Haynes R B. Of studies，syntheses，synopses，summaries，and systems：the "5S" evolution of information services for evidence-based health care decisions. Acp Journal Club，2005，145(3)：A8.

（2）Haynes R B. Of studies，summaries，synopses，and systems：the "4S" evolution of services for finding current best evidence. Acp Journal Club，2001，134(2)：A11.

（3）Dicenso A，Bayley L，Haynes R B. Accessing pre-appraised evidence：Fine tuning 5S model into the 6S model. Evidence Based Nursing，2009，151(6)：99-101.

第二部分　教学设计——4课时（160分钟）

"证据检索"教学设计表

序号	内　容	互动技术/教学技术	描　　　述	时间（分钟）
1	检索证据的基本步骤	PPT 演示	向学生简单介绍检索证据的基本步骤	5
2	第一步：定义临床问题	PPT 演示	复习用于构建临床问题的 PICO 格式	3
3	第二步：选择最合适的数据库	PPT 演示 互动 4.1：创造性会话	请学生们阅读有关 6S 模型的阅读资料，然后互相交流 6S 模型中每个"S"的意思、代表什么、我们应该如何运用 6S 模型	17
4	第三步：构建检索策略	PPT 演示 互动 4.2：拼字 互动 4.3：头脑风暴	Scrabble：用医学术语"cancer（癌）"作为例子，请学生们将其同义词和近义词列举出来。头脑风暴：让学生们思考如何才能尽可能全面地把有关癌的文献都检索出来，引出主题词概念和主题词检索方法	15
5	第四步：构建检索策略——MeSH	PPT 演示	引出 MeSH 这一有用的检索途径	12
6	第五步：构建检索策略——MeSH 和关键词的优缺点	互动 4.4：利弊面 PPT 演示	应用利弊面技术请学生们思考 MeSH 和关键词的优缺点并请两名学生将其列在黑板上，然后运用 PPT 将优缺点列出并与学生列出的结果进行比较	15
7	第六步：构建检索策略——检索策略的基本结构	PPT 演示	介绍检索策略的基本结构，其中用到布尔逻辑运算符	13

（续表）

序号	内　容	互动技术/教学技术	描　　　述	时间（分钟）
8	案例	PPT 演示	向学生们演示在具体案例中怎样一步一步地构建检索策略	15
9	练习	PPT 演示 互动 4.5：传递问题	将学生分成 5 个组,给学生们一个案例,请第一组学生回答第一个问题(约 3 分钟),请下一组学生识别下一个问题,直到 5 个问题回答完毕。	25
10	常用数据库	PPT 演示、实际操作演示	演示常用数据库的使用	25
11	实践	互动 4.6：实践与评价	请学生们对互动 4.5 中出现的案例实际进行检索,找出循证医学证据	15

第三部分　教　学　内　容

1. 证据检索的基本步骤

（1）定义临床问题。
（2）选择最合适的数据库。
（3）构建检索策略。
（4）评估证据。

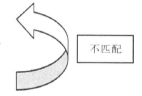

不匹配

2. 定义临床问题

临床问题引导我们进行检索。在前面的章节中我们讨论了怎样运用 PICO 格式来构建临床问题：

P＝population/patient/problem（人群/患者/问题）

I＝intervention/diagnostic test/prognostic factor/exposure
　　（干预/诊断试验/预后/暴露因素）

C＝comparison（对照）

O＝outcome（结局）

3. 选择合适的数据库

近年来,支持循证临床决策的资源发展迅速。在迅速发展的临床重大研究、系统评价和证据摘要，以及迅猛发展的信息技术和信息系统的推动下，更新、更好的证据服务层出不穷。为此，Haynes 引入了 6S 证据系统来帮助我们选择合适的资源。

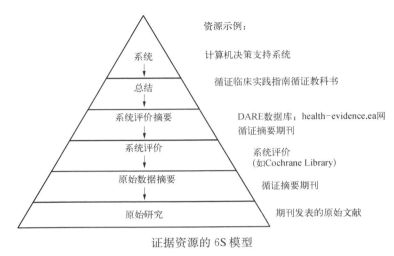

证据资源的 6S 模型

总的原则：优先选择二次研究证据源，次选原始研究证据源。

我们应该从证据模型的最高级开始选择数据库，若没有找到合适的证据，再逐级往下选择数据库进行检索，直到找到合适的证据。

互动 4.1：创造性会话

教师：现在请同学们阅读材料。

（1）Haynes R B. Of studies，syntheses，synopses，summaries，and systems：the "5S" evolution of information services for evidence-based health care decisions. Acp Journal Club，2005，145(3)：A8.

（2）Haynes R B. Of studies，summaries，synopses，and systems：the "4S" evolution of services for finding current best evidence. Acp Journal Club，2001，134(2)：A11.

（3）Dicenso A，Bayley L，Haynes R B. Accessing pre-appraised evidence：Fine tuning 5S model into the 6S model. Evidence Based Nursing，2009，151(6)：99－101.

然后互相交流 6S 模型中每个 "S" 的意思、代表什么以及我们应该怎样运用 6S 模型。

学生：（交流）

4. 构建检索策略

首先,我们应该从已经构建的临床问题的四个要素中抽取检索词,同时这些要素还可以帮助我们找到相应的同义词。

要构建合适的检索策略,首先我们需要了解两种常用的检索途径——主题词和关键词。

互动 4.2: 拼字

教师: 癌是一类我们非常熟悉的学习过的疾病。当我们要检索与癌相关的证据时,不同的作者会选择不同的癌的表达方式来撰写论文。现在,请大家列出"cancer(癌)"的同义词。

学生 1: Neoplasm.

学生 2: Tumor.

学生 3: Carcinoma.

教师: 非常好,这些都是医学术语"cancer"的同义词或近义词。当我们撰写论文时,我们可能会用其中的任一个词;当我们检索时,我们也会使用任意一个词。但是,如果我们使用了不同的词来进行检索,我们会获得不同的检索结果。

互动 4.3: 头脑风暴

教师: 假设大家是癌症领域的研究者,每位同学都发表过相关文章,而大家所使用的癌的表述不一样(可能是我们在互动 4.2 中列举的任一个)。怎样能尽可能全面地检索到大家的文章呢?

(数分钟后)

学生 1: 尽可能检索更多的数据库.

学生 2: 对所有它的同义词和近义词进行检索

学生 3: 我们之前学习了 MeSH,我们可以使用 MeSH 来检索

教师: 非常好,大家已经想到了一些常用的查全的方法。

5. MeSH

MeSH 的全名是医学主题词,是美国国家医学图书馆推出的规范化的词表。该表由一套叫做"主题词"的术语组成,这些主题词有树状结构,这个结构允许我们对主题词进行扩检和缩检。

在主题词表中，主题词有两种排列的方式，一种是按照字母顺序进行排列，另一种是按照树状结构进行排列。在树状结构中，最大级别的是含义较宽的主题词，如解剖学、精神异常。级别越低的词汇，其含义范围越窄、越精确，如踝、行为障碍。在主题词表中，有超过 2.9 万个主题词及超过 10 万个主题词的入口词，这些入口词可以帮助我们找到最合适的主题词。例如，"cancer（癌）"是"neoplasms（肿瘤）"的入口词。在常用的数据库中，Cochrane Library 和 PubMed 提供主题词检索途径。

6. MeSH 和关键词检索的优缺点

互动 4.4：利弊面

教师： 请大家思考几分钟有关 MeSH 和关键词的优缺点并把它们写在黑板上。

（数分钟后）

学生 1： MeSH 优点是它是规范化的。

学生 2： MeSH 优点是它可以和副主题词搭配检索。

学生 3： MeSH 缺点是不能自由使用。

学生 4： 关键词使用起来比较自由。

学生 5： 当我们使用关键词检索而没能列全同义词时，可能会有文献漏检。

教师： 很好，我们在检索时应该根据我们选择的数据库的特点以及我们的检索需求来选择检索途径。

7. 检索策略的基本结构

当我们把问题拆分为 PICO 几个元素后，我们就能将它们用布尔逻辑运算符"AND"和"OR"连接起来进行检索：

P（患者 OR 同义词 1 OR 同义词 2……）AND

I（干预措施 OR 同义词 1 OR 同义词 2……）AND

C（对照 OR 同义词 1 OR 同义词 2……）AND

O（结局 OR 同义词 1 OR 同义词 2……）AND

布尔逻辑运算符包括 AND、OR、NOT。它们能帮助我们扩大或者缩小检索范围。使用 AND 能帮助我们检索到输入的所有检索词，如"心脏骤停"AND"经皮冠状动脉介入术"找到的是同时具有短语"心脏骤停"和短语"经皮冠状动脉介入术"的文章。OR 能帮助我们找到包含指定单词或短语中的任一个的研究。例如,"心脏骤停"OR"经皮冠状动脉介入"找到的是具有短语"心脏骤停"或短语"经皮冠状动脉介入"的文章。NOT 排除包含指定单词或短语的文章。例如,"心脏骤停"NOT"经皮冠状动脉介入术",找到的是含有短语"心脏骤停"但不含有短语"经皮冠状动脉介入术"的文章。

将问题的所有四个元素(PICO)结合在一起来检索,可能导致检索到的文章很少甚至没有。如果这样,我们应该重新设计我们的检索策略。通常,"P"和"I"部分是检索的必要部分,我们是否使用其他两个组件来构建检索策略需要根据具体情况来决定。

8. 案例

Jack 是一位 35 岁成年人,既往史无特殊,因咳嗽、咯痰 2 天来就诊。你的初步诊断是急性支气管炎。

我们都知道急性支气管炎可能由病毒或细菌引起。在很多诊所里抗生素常被用于这种情况,但是你对此持怀疑态度。

现在他的实验室检查结果未回,你想要知道使用抗生素是否有益?

我们在检索循证医学证据时有一些问题是值得我们关注的。

(1)定义一个可检索的问题

P：患急性支气管炎的成人

I：抗生素

C：安慰剂/空白对照

O：使用抗生素的有效性和安全性

(2)最合适的数据库：根据我们前面学习的 6S 模型,我们应该从 6S 的最顶端选择数据库开始进行检索。

(3)问题的类型：这是什么类型的问题?(治疗/诊断/病因/预后/不良反应)这是治疗性问题。

(4)证据类型：对这种类型的问题哪种证据是最佳的? 基于随机对照试验的系统评价或随机对照试验

(5)检索策略

A. 主题词途径：acute bronchitis/drug therapy[MeSH] and antibiotic/therapuetic use[MeSH].

B. 关键词检索：acute bronchitis and (antibiotic or anti bacterial agents or anti-bacterial compounds or bacteriocidal agents or antibiotic …).

9. 练习

互动 4.5：传递问题

将学生进行分组，针对以下临床情境回答问题，第一组回答第一个问题（3分钟），将问题传到下一组并请他们找出下一个问题的答案。以此类推直至所有问题都被回答了。

分析下列情境并回答问题：

Jim 是一位 19 岁男孩，患有 IgA 肾病，合并有高血压和蛋白尿。现在我们想知道血管紧张素抑制剂（ACEI）是否能延缓其病程。

教师：现在请同学们从 1 到 10 进行报数。（这里我们将学生分为 5 组，如果需要 8 组则从 1 到 8 进行报数，我们假设全班有 50 名学生。）请同学们记住自己的报数数字。

学生：（报数）

教师：现在所有报数为 1 的同学为 1 组，报数为 2 的为 2 组，报数为 3 的为 3 组……

问题 1，定义一个可检索的问题

1 组：P：IgA 肾病；I：血管紧张素抑制剂（ACEI）；C：安慰剂/标准治疗；O：延缓病程。

教师：很好！问题 2，最合适的数据库呢？

2 组：Cochrane Library

教师：很好！问题 3，这是什么类型的问题？（治疗/诊断/病因/预后/不良反应）

3 组：这是治疗性问题。

教师：很好！问题 4，对这种类型的问题哪种证据是最佳的证据类型？

4 组：基于随机对照试验的系统评价或随机对照试验

教师：很好！问题 5，你们的检索策略是什么？

5 组：我们使用主题词检索：IgA nephropathy/drug therapy[MeSH] and angiotensin converting enzyme inhibitor/therapuetic use[MeSH]。

10. 常用免费数据库的使用

（1）Cochrane Library：主页为 http://www.cochranelibrary.com/（更多信息可参见 http://www.cochranelibrary.com/help/how-to-use-cochrane-library.html）。

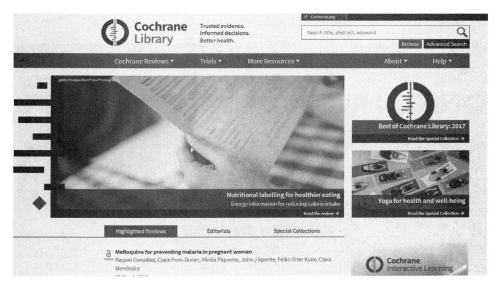

Cochrane Library 主页

Cochrane Library 是一个数据库集合，其中包含不同类型的高质量独立证据来为医疗决策提供证据。

Cochrane Library 概况

数 据 库	内 容
Cochrane 系统评价数据库（CDSR）	CDSR 是卫生保健领域系统评价的主要来源。CDSR 中的文献类型包括 Cochrane 系统评价、Cochrane 系统评价的协议、社论和补充材料（包括 Cochrane 会议摘要和 Cochrane 方法学的内容）
Cochrane 中心对照试验注册中心（CENTRAL）	Central 高度集中了随机和半随机对照试验。其中大多数记录来自书目数据库（主要是 PubMed 和 Embase），也有记录来自其他已出版和未出版的来源，包括美国临床试验数据库（Clinical Trials.gov）和世界卫生组织国际临床试验注册平台（International Clinical Trials Registry Platform）
Cochrane 临床答案（CCAs）	CCAs 提供了一个可读性强、易懂、以临床为中心的来源于 Cochrane 系统评价的严谨研究的入口。每个 Cochrane 临床答案都包含一个临床问题、一个简短的答案和 Cochrane 系统评价的结果数据

资料来源：http://www.cochranelibrary.com/about/about-the-cochrane-library.html

以上资源均可在 Cochrane Library 主页找到。

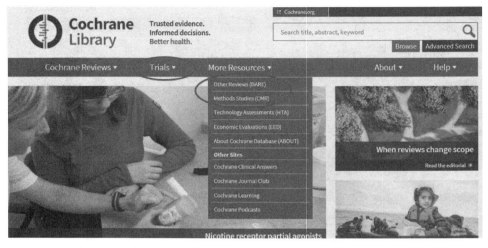

Cochrane Library 资源

　　A. 简单检索：直接在检索框中输入检索词并点击检索按钮，就可得到检索结果。

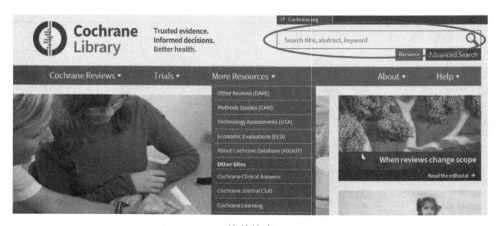

简单检索

　　B. 高级检索

● 点击高级检索按钮来进行更复杂的检索，也可由此进入检索编辑器及主题词检索。

● 高级检索页面：从检索选项卡中，使用菜单选项限定检索字段，如全文、

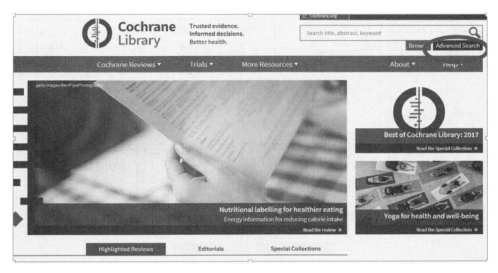

高级检索按钮

标题、作者、摘要或关键字。高级检索支持通用搜索语法：布尔运算符（AND、OR、NOT）、位置运算符（NEAR、NEXT）和截词符（＊、？）。

● 检索编辑器：检索编辑器可以帮助我们构建复杂的检索策略。

C. 主题词检索：点击"Medical Terms（MeSH）"选项即可进入主题词检索页面。

D. 结果页面。

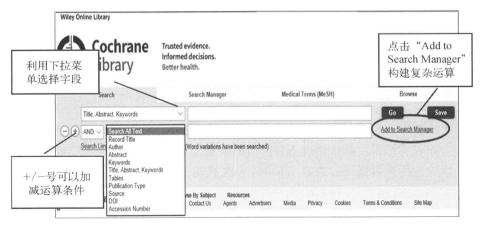

高级检索页面

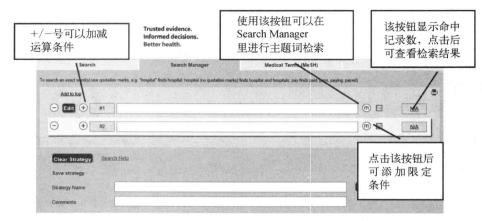

检索编辑器

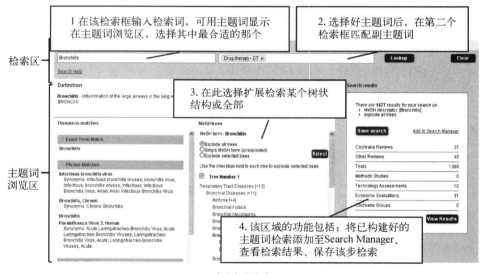

主题词检索

- 按数据库查看结果：在结果页面中，可以使用单选按钮（"radio"）按数据库查看结果。默认情况下，除非使用"搜索限定"选项进行了限定，否则将检索所有数据库。查看结果时，一次只能选择一个数据库。括号中的数字是为该数据库检索的文章数量。
- 检索结果排序：可将检索结果按相关度、标题字顺或日期排序。默认按相关度排序。

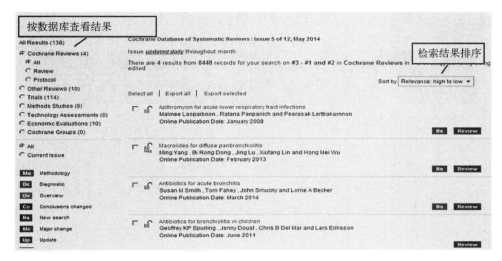

检索结果页面

（2）PubMed：主页为 https://www.ncbi.nlm.nih.gov/pubmed/。

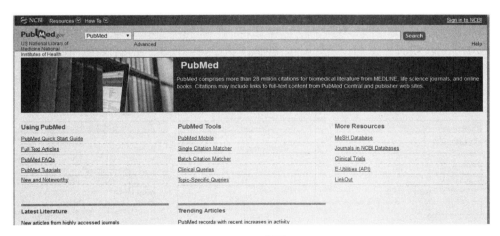

PubMed 主页

PubMed 包含超过 2 800 万条来自 MEDLINE、*Life Science Journals* 和在线的生物医学文献的记录。这些记录可提供来自 PubMed Central 和发布网站的全文内容的链接。PubMed 是美国国立卫生研究院的美国国家医学图书馆的美国国家生物技术信息中心（NCBI）开发和维护的免费资源。

A. 临床查询：临床查询是旨在检索针对临床问题的结果的搜索工具。可以从 PubMed 主页访问临床查询。

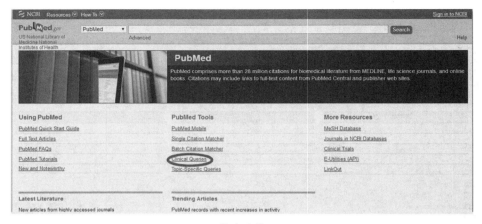

临床查询

在临床查询中，可以输入检索词并单击检索按钮。在结果页面中，显示前 5 个检索到的记录。结果页面有三个过滤器：临床研究类别、系统评价和医学遗传学。其中临床研究类型过滤器可以按类别检索，找到与特定主题的病因、诊断、治疗或预后特别相关的文章，还可扩大和缩小检索范围。系统评价过滤器允许检索 Meta 分析、临床实验系统综述和循证医学指南。医学遗传学过滤器查找与医学遗传学各种主题相关的记录，如临床描述、基因检测和鉴别诊断的内容。

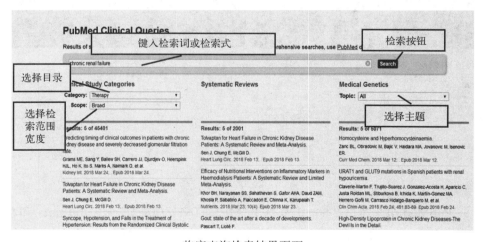

临床查询检索结果页面

B. 直接在 PubMed 检索循证医学证据：如果在检索策略中有任何其他限定条件，可以直接在 PubMed 中检索，并使用结果页面中的过滤器来进行限定，如日期、语言、文献类型等。

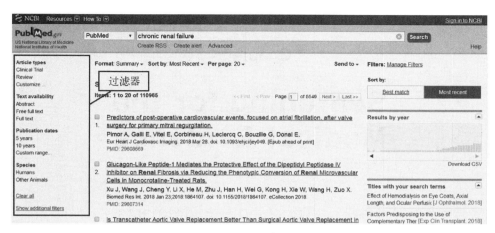

PubMed 过滤器

互动 4.6：实践与评价

【案例】Jack 是一位 35 岁成年人，既往史无特殊，因咳嗽、咯痰 2 天就诊。你的初步诊断是急性支气管炎。

我们都知道急性支气管炎可能由病毒或细菌引起。在很多诊所里抗生素常被用于这种情况，但是你对此持怀疑态度。

现在他的实验室检查结果未回，你想要知道抗生素是否有益？

教师：请每个组的同学都再次思考以上案例、编写你们的检索策略并使用我们刚刚介绍的数据库进行检索。我们将请 1 到 2 组同学演示他们如何得到的证据，其他组同学对他们的检索进行评价。

（数分钟后）

1 组和 2 组：（演示）

3 组：（评价）

4 组：（评价）

5 组：（评价）

谭睿璟

Chapter 4

Searching for the Medical Evidence

Part I　Teaching Requirements

This teaching session is mainly about the steps of evidence retrieval, including the discussion of each step, introduction to the use of common databases and the practice of retrieval.

1. Teaching aims

To learn and practice the basic steps of acquiring evidence and common evidence-based medicine information sources.

2. Learning objectives

After completing this session, students should be able to:
(1) Understand the 6S approach of evidence resources.
(2) Apply the basic steps of acquiring evidence.
(3) Retrieve evidence from the common EBM information sources such as Cochrane Library and PubMed.

3. Teaching methods

This session will use lecture, PPT presentation and interactive teaching method. Interactive teaching techniques include, invented dialogues, scrabble, brainstorming, pro and con grid, and pass the problem.

4. Reading materials

(1) Haynes R B. Of studies, syntheses, synopses, summaries, and systems: the "5S" evolution of information services for evidence-based health

care decisions. Acp Journal Club, 2005, 145(3): A8.

(2) Haynes R B. Of studies, summaries, synopses, and systems: the "4S" evolution of services for finding current best evidence. Acp Journal Club, 2001, 134(2): A11.

(3) Dicenso A, Bayley L, Haynes R B. Accessing pre-appraised evidence: Fine tuning 5S model into the 6S model. Evidence Based Nursing, 2009, 151(6): 99 – 101.

Part II　Teaching Design — 4 periods（160 minutes）

Teaching design of "Searching for the Medical Evidence"

No.	Content	Interactive technique/ teaching techniques	Descriptions	Time （minutes）
1	Basic steps of searching for evidence	PPT presentation	Generally introduce the basic steps of searching for evidence to the students.	5
2	Step 1: Defining a clinical question	PPT presentation	Review the PICO format of building questions.	3
3	Step 2: Selecting the most appropriate resource	PPT presentation Interaction 4.1: Invented dialogues	Ask students to read the reading materials, and then make them weave together quotes from these materials about what each "S" stands for, the meaning of each "S" and how we can use the 6S approach.	17
4	Step 3: Building search strategy	PPT presentation Interaction 4.2: Scrabble Interaction 4.3: Brainstorming	**Scrabble:** Use the medical terminology "cancer" as the example, ask the students to list as many synonyms of it as possible. (For example, neoplasm, tumor, carcinoma, etc.). **Brainstorming:** Students think about how to search for articles as many as possible related to cancer. The method is used to get students to focus on using MeSH term to search for evidence.	15

（continued）

No.	Content	Interactive techniques/ teaching techniques	Descriptions	Time (minutes)
5	Step 4：Building search strategy — MeSH	PPT presentation	Introduce MeSH headings which is a useful way to search.	12
6	Step 5：Building search strategy — advantages and disadvantages of MeSH and key words	Interaction 4.4：Pro and con grid PPT presentation	Ask students to think for a few minutes about the pro & con of MeSH and the key words and list them on the board. Then show the pro & con by PPT and compare them with the pro & con listed by students.	15
7	Step 6：Building search strategy — basic structure of search strategy	PPT presentation	Introduce the basic structure of search strategy using Boolean operators.	13
8	Scenario	PPT presentation	Show students how to manage a search strategy step by step with a scenario.	15
9	Practice	PPT presentation Interaction 4.5：Pass the problem	Divide the students into 5 groups. Give the students a case，ask the first group to answer the first question （3 minutes）. Pass the problems on to the next group and have them identify the next problem. Continue until all the questions have been answered.	25
10	Commonly used database	PPT presentation Practical demonstration	Introduce the use of popular database.	25
11	Practice	Interaction 4.6：Practice and assessment	Ask students to search for the evidence in the above case in Interaction 4.5 in groups.	15

Part III　Teaching Contents

1. Basic steps of searching for evidence

（1）Defining a clinical question.

（2）Selecting the most appropriate resource.

（3）Designing search strategy.

（4）Appraising the evidence.

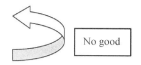

No good

2. Defining a clinical question

The question guides the search. We have discussed how to formulate an answerable question with PICO format in the previous chapter. Here：

P＝population/patient/problem

I＝intervention/diagnostic test/prognostic factor/exposure

C＝comparison

O＝outcome

3. Select the most appropriate resource

Practical resources to support evidence-based clinical decisions are rapidly evolving. New and better services are being created through the combined force of the increasing number of clinically important studies, more evidence synthesis and synopsis service, and better information technology and systems. Haynes introduced a 6S approach to help us choose the appropriate resource.

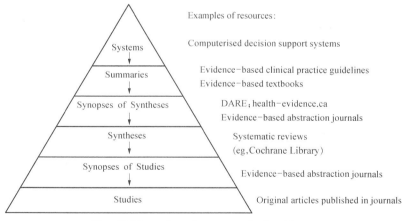

The 6S hierarchy of pre-appraised evidence

A general rule：select evidence resources of secondary research first, then primary sources.

We should begin with our search for best evidence by looking at the highest-level resource available for the problem that prompts your search. If a suitable database is not found, we should select databases step by step to search, untill we find the most suitable one.

Interaction 4.1： Invented dialogues

Teacher：Please read the reading material：

（1）Haynes R B. Of studies, syntheses, synopses, summaries, and systems：the "5S" evolution of information services for evidence-based health care decisions. Acp Journal Club, 2005, 145(3)：A8.

（2）Haynes R B. Of studies, summaries, synopses, and systems：the "4S" evolution of services for finding current best evidence. Acp Journal Club, 2001, 134(2)：A11.

（3）Dicenso A, Bayley L, Haynes R B. Accessing pre-appraised evidence：Fine tuning 5S model into the 6S model. Evidence Based Nursing, 2009, 151(6)：99 - 101.

Then weave together quotes from these materials about what each "s" stands for, the meaning of each "s" and how we can use the 6s approach.

Students：(communicating)

---

4. Designing search strategy

First, we should extract search terms from the four elements of the constructed clinical question, which can also help us find synonyms.

To design a proper search strategy, we need to understand MeSH term and key word — two commonly-used search ways.

Interaction 4.2： Scrabble

Teacher：Cancer is a kind of disease we have all heard of and learnt about. When we search evidence of cancer, we will find out that different author would prefer different words to write their articles. Now please list as many synonyms of it as possible.

Student 1：Neoplasm.

Student 2：Tumor.

Student 3：Carcinoma.

Teacher：Very good, these are all synonyms of the medical terminology "cancer", when we write articles, we may use any of them; when we search, we also can do so. But if we choose different search words, we will get different results.

Interaction 4.3 : Brainstorming

Teacher: Suppose you are scholars in the domain of cancer research, and each of you has published an article about this disease while the exact words used in your article are different — which could be any word we have listed in Interaction 4.2. Now how can we get as many articles as possible?

(several minutes later)

Student 1: Search as many databases as possible.

Student 2: Use all the synonyms to search.

Student 3: We have studied MeSH before; we can use MeSH to search.

Teacher: Very good, you have listed several commonly used ways to solve this problem.

5. MeSH

The full name of MeSH is Medical Subject Headings and it is a standardized glossary published by National Library of Medicine of the United States. It consists of sets of terms, namely, descriptors in a hierarchical structure that permits searching at various levels of specificity.

MeSH descriptors are arranged in both an alphabetic and a hierarchical structure. At the most general level of the hierarchical structure are the broader headings such as "anatomy" or "mental disorders." More specific headings are found at more narrow levels, such as "ankle" and "conduct disorder." There are over 29,000 descriptors in MeSH with over 100,000 entry terms that assist in finding the most appropriate MeSH. For example, "cancer" is an entry term to "neoplasms." MeSH is available on PubMed and Cochrane Library.

6. Pro and con grid of MeSH and key word

Interaction 4.4 : Pro and con grid

Teacher: Please think for a few minutes about the pro and con of MeSH and the key word and list them on the board.

（several minutes later）

Student 1: Advantage of MeSH: it is standard.

Student 2: Advantage of MeSH: it can work with subheadings.

Student 3: Disadvantage of MeSH: can not be used freely.

Student 4: Key word is more flexible.

Student 5: If we use a key word to search, and if we can not find out all the synonyms, we can easily miss articles.

Teacher: Very good. When we search, we should choose the search fields depending on the database we are using and the need of searching.

7. Basic structure of search strategy

Once the study question has been broken down into its components, they can be combined by using the Boolean operators "AND" and "OR":

P（population OR synonym 1 OR synonym 2 ...）And

I（intervention OR synonym 1 OR synonym 2 ...）And

C（comparison OR synonym 1 OR synonym 2 ...）And

O（outcome OR synonym 1 OR synonym 2 ...）And

Boolean operators are AND, OR and NOT. They can broaden or narrow our search results. AND finds studies containing all specified words or phrases. For example, "cardiac arrest" AND "percutaneous coronary intervention" finds articles with both the phrase "cardiac arrest" and the phrase "percutaneous coronary intervention". OR finds studies containing either of the specified words or phrases. For example, "cardiac arrest" OR "percutaneous coronary intervention" finds articles with either the phrase "cardiac arrest" or the phrase "percutaneous coronary intervention". NOT excludes studies containing the specified word or phrase. For example, "cardiac arrest" NOT "percutaneous coronary intervention" finds articles with the phrase "cardiac arrest" but not the phrase "percutaneous coronary intervention".

There's a chance that combing all of the four components of questions together may result in few or even no articles. Then we should redesign our search strategy. Usually, the "P" and "I" parts are the necessary ones of the four components,. Whether we use the other two components to design our search strategy depends on the situation.

8. Scenario

Jack is a 35-year-old adult whose medical history was unremarkable; he has been coughing with sputum for two days. He comes to the clinic asking for help. You give him a diagnosis of acute bronchitis.

You know acute bronchitis may be caused by viruses or bacteria. Antibiotics are commonly prescribed to treat this condition in most clinics, but you doubt it.

Now the results of his laboratory examinations are not available yet, so you want to know whether antibiotics are beneficial or not?

There are some questions we should focus on when we search:

(1) Define a searchable question

P: adult suffering from acute bronchitis.

I: antibiotics.

C: placebo/no treatment.

O: effects and safety of using antibiotics.

(2) The most likely source: According to the 6S approach we have discussed before, we should begin with our search at the highest possible layer in the 6S model.

(3) The type of question: What kind of question is this (therapy/diagnostic/etiology/prognosis/harm)? It is about therapy.

(4) The type of evidence: What type of evidence is suggested for this kind of question? Systematic review based on RCTs or RCTs.

(5) Our search strategy

A. through MeSH: acute bronchitis/drug therapy [MeSH] and antibiotic/therapuetic use[MeSH].

B. through key word: acute bronchitis and (antibiotic or Anti Bacterial Agents or Anti-Bacterial Compounds or Bacteriocidal Agents or antibiotic ...).

9. Practice

Interaction 4.5 : Pass the problem
Classify students into groups. Give the students the following case,

and ask the first group to answer the first question（3 minutes）. Pass the problem onto the next group and have them identify the next step. Continue until all groups have contributed.

Read the following scenario. Then please finish the answer：

Jim is a 19-year-old boy suffering from IgA nephropathy with hypertension and proteinuria. We want to know whether the drug angiotensin converting enzyme inhibitor（ACEI）could be used to slow down his progression.

Teacher：Now I need you to call out number from 1 to 10 one by one.（Here we divide the students into 5 groups，if we need 8 groups，call out from 1 to 8，and so on. The number of the students in the class is assumed as 50.）Please be sure to remember the number of yourself.

Students：（call out the number）

Teacher：Now，all number 1 students go together to be a group；all number 2s a group，all number 3s a group …

Question 1，define a searchable question.

Group 1：P：IgA nephropathy；I：angiotensin converting enzyme inhibitor（ACEI）；C：placebo/standard treatment；O：slow down the progression.

Teacher：Good！ Question 2，which database is suitable and available?

Group 2：Cochrane Library.

Teacher：Good！ Question 3，what kind of question is this?（therapy/diagnostic/etiology/prognosis/harm）

Group 3：Therapy.

Teacher：Good！ Question 4，what type of evidence is suggested for this kind of question?

Group 4：Systematic review based on SRs or RCTs.

Teacher：Good！ Question 5，your search strategy?

Group 5：We use MeSH to search：IgA nephropathy/drug therapy ［MeSH］and angiotensin converting enzyme inhibitor/therapuetic use ［MeSH］.

10. The use of common free databases

(1) Cochrane Library: The homepage is http://www.cochranelibrary. com/. (More information can be found at: http://www.cochranelibrary. com/help/how-to-use-cochrane-library.html.)

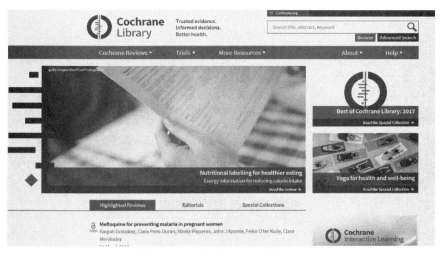

Homepage of Cochrane Library

The Cochrane Library is a collection of databases that contain different types of high-quality, independent evidence to inform researchers of medical decisions.

Overview of Cochrane Library

Database	Content
Cochrane Database of Systematic Reviews (CDSR)	CDSR is the leading resource for systematic reviews in health care. CDSR includes Cochrane reviews (systematic reviews) and protocols for Cochrane reviews as well as editorials and supplements (including abstracts of Cochrane colloquia and other conferences and Cochrane methods).
Cochrane Central Register of Controlled Trials (CENTRAL)	CENTRAL is a highly concentrated source of reports of randomized and quasi-randomized controlled trials. Most CENTRAL records are taken from bibliographic databases (mainly PubMed and Embase), some records are also derived from other published and unpublished sources, including ClinicalTrials.gov and the WHO's International Clinical Trials Registry Platform.

(continued)

Database	Content
Cochrane Clinical Answers（CCAs）	CCAs provide a readable，digestible，clinically-focused entry point to rigorous research from Cochrane Reviews. Each CCA contains a clinical question，a short answer，and data for the outcomes from the Cochrane Review.

（resource from：http://www.cochranelibrary.com/about/about-the-cochrane-library.html）

All the sources above could be found on the homepage.

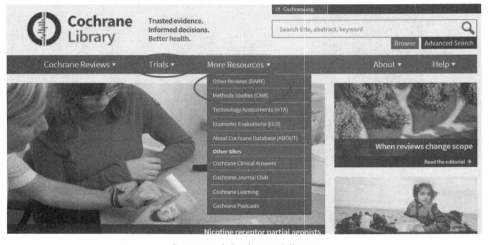

Sources of Cochrane Library

A. Simple search：Type a search term directly into the search box and click the search button and we can get the result.

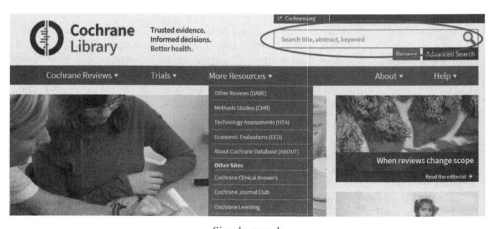

Simple search

B. Advanced search:

● Select "Advanced Search" to create complex searches. Go into the search manager or search by MeSH.

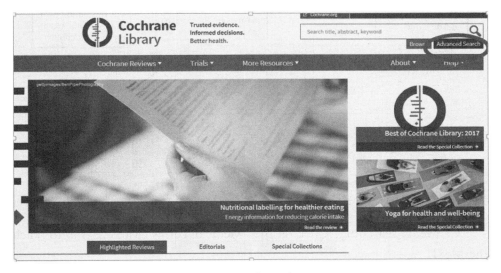

Advanced search

● The advanced search page: From the search tab, use the menu selection to easily limit searches to the fields, such as full text, title, author, abstract or keywords. It supports common search syntax: Boolean operators (AND, OR, NOT), proximity operators (NEAR, NEXT) and truncation (*,?).

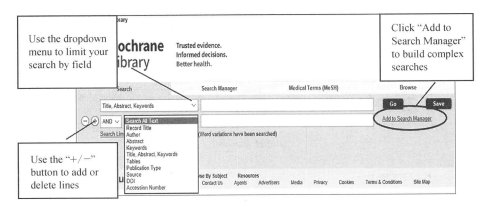

Advanced search

● Search Manager：The search manager helps us to create complex search strategies.

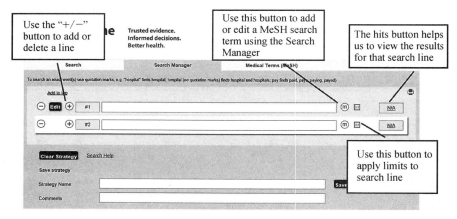

Use the "+/−" button to add or delete a line

Use this button to add or edit a MeSH search term using the Search Manager

The hits button helps us to view the results for that search line

Use this button to apply limits to search line

Search manager

C. MeSH searching：Click on the "Medical Terms（MeSH）" tab to reach the MeSH search page.

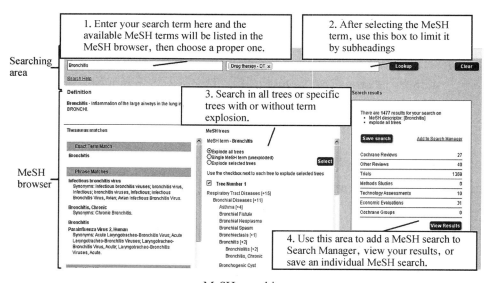

1. Enter your search term here and the available MeSH terms will be listed in the MeSH browser, then choose a proper one.

2. After selecting the MeSH term, use this box to limit it by subheadings

3. Search in all trees or specific trees with or without term explosion.

4. Use this area to add a MeSH search to Search Manager, view your results, or save an individual MeSH search.

MeSH searching

D. Result page：

● View results by database：In the result page，we can view results by database using the "radio" button. By default，all databases are searched unless restrictions have been made using the "Search Limits" option. When we view results, only one database can be selected at a time. Number in parentheses is the number of articles retrieved for that database.

● Sort results: We also can sort results by relevance, title, or data, or in alphabetical order. Default sort is by relevance.

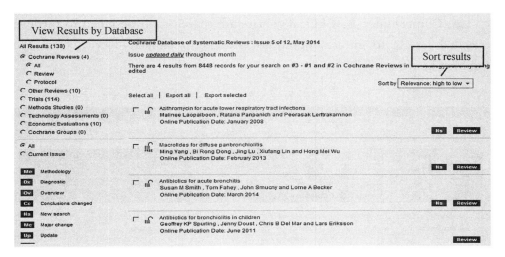

Result page

(2) PubMed: The homepage is https://www.ncbi.nlm.nih.gov/pubmed/.

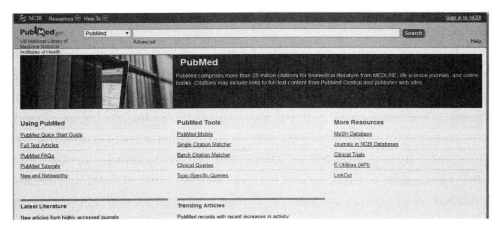

Homepage of PubMed

PubMed comprises more than 28 million citations for biomedical literatures from MEDLINE，*Life Science Journals*，and online books. Citations may include links to full-text content from PubMed Central and publisher web sites. PubMed is a free resource that is developed and maintained by National Center for Biotechnology Information（NCBI），at National Library of Medicine（NLM），located at National Institutes of Health（NIH）.

A. Clinical queries：Clinical queries are search tools designed to retrieve targeted results to clinical questions. Access to clinical queries from the PubMed homepage.

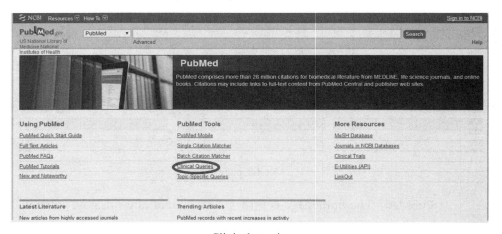

Clinical queries

In clinical queries，we can enter our search term（s）and click search button. In the result page，the first 5 retrieved citations are displayed. There are three filters：clinical study categories，systematic reviews and medical genetics. We can search by clinical study category to find articles specifically related to etiology，diagnosis，therapy or prognosis of a specific topic and use the scope button to broaden or narrow the results. Systematic review filter allows a searcher to find citations for meta-analysis，reviews of clinical trails，evidence-based medicine，and guidelines. Medical genetics filter finds citations related to various topics in medical genetics，such as clinical description，genetic testing，and differential diagnosis.

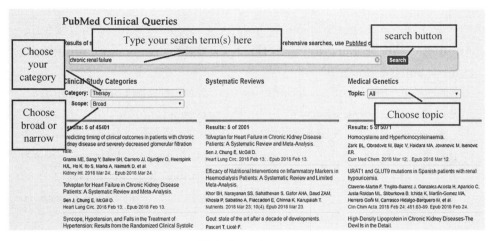

Clinical queries page

B. Search directly in PubMed: If there is any other limits in our search strategy, we can also search directly in PubMed, using the filters existing in the result page to set limits such as dates, languages, article types, and so on.

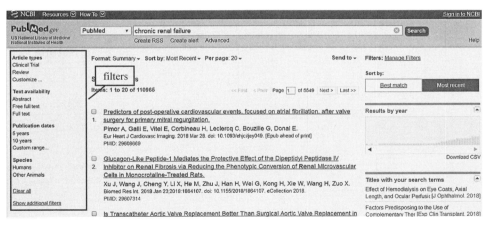

PubMed result filters

Interaction 4.6 : Practice and assessment

【Case】Jack is a 35-year-old adult whose medical history was unremarkable, he has been coughing with sputum for two days. He comes to the clinic asking for help. You give him a diagnosis of acute bronchitis.

You know acute bronchitis may be caused by viruses or bacteria. Antibiotics are commonly prescribed to treat this condition in most clinics, but you doubt it.

Now the results of his laboratory examinations are not available yet, so you want to know whether antibiotics are beneficial or not?

Teacher: We have discussed the case twice. Now, please consider it again, build your search strategy and apply it to the database we just learned. Find evidence to support your position. Then we'll have 1 or 2 groups to demonstrate how they get the evidence, and other groups to assess their searching performances.

(several minutes later)

Group 1 and group 2: (demonstrate)

Group 3: (assess)

Group 4: (assess)

Group 5: (assess)

Tan Ruijing

第 5 章

临床实践中的患者价值观

第一部分　教　学　要　求

循证医学强调最佳证据、医生素养和患者价值观的结合,因此如何在个体患者的临床决策中有效地融合患者的价值观及意愿选择,是循证医学发展面临的重要挑战。希望通过本章的学习,学生能够掌握患者价值观的定义、差异性特点及局限性;熟悉常用的循证决策辅助工具和共同决策模式(SDM);了解如何在实践中正确地引导患者的价值观。

1. 教学目的

掌握价值观与意愿的定义和意义,并能够运用决策辅助系统和共同决策模式帮助患者制定诊疗方案。

2. 学习目标

通过此环节的学习,学生能够:
(1) 描述患者价值观与意愿的定义、差异性特点及局限性。
(2) 描述常用的循证决策辅助工具和医患共同决策模式(SDM)。
(3) 选择合适的方法在实践中引导患者的价值观。

3. 教学方法

此环节采用讲授法、PPT 演示和互动教学法。互动教学技术包括思考时段、苏格拉底式提问和门诊角色扮演等教学法。

4. 阅读材料

(1) Alonso-Coello P，Montori V M，Díaz M G，et al. Values and preferences for oral antithrombotic therapy in patients with atrial fibrillation：physician and patient perspectives. Health Expect.，2015，18(6)：2318 - 2327.

（2）Maclean S，Mulla S，Akl E A，et al. Patient values and preferences in decision making for antithrombotic therapy：a systematic review：antithrombotic therapy and prevention of thrombosis，9th ed：American college of chest physicians evidence-based clinical practice guidelines. Chest，2012，141(2)：e1S-23S.

第二部分　教学设计——2 课时（80 分钟）

"临床实践中的患者价值观"教学设计表

序号	内　容	互动技术/教学技术	描　　　　述	时间（分钟）
1	患者价值观定义、差异性特点	PPT 演示 互动 5.1：思考时段	通过 PPT 向学生们展示案例，令其思考并与同桌讨论，其后介绍 Gordon Guyatt 提出的定义	10
2	患者价值观的重要性和局限性	互动 5.2：苏格拉底式提问	教师通过一系列设问，引出患者价值观的差异性特点、重要性及其在临床诊疗决策中的局限性	30
3	临床决策模式	PPT 演示	临床决策模式及共同决策模式应注意的几个方面	15
4	患者辅助决策工具	PPT 演示	以证据为基础，帮助患者详细了解不同治疗方案的益处和风险，平衡患者的综合需求	5
5	共同决策模式实践（SDM）	互动 5.3：门诊角色扮演	通过门诊角色扮演让学生们领会患者价值观在临床决策中的作用、熟悉共同决策模式	20

第三部分　教　学　内　容

1. 患者价值观定义

互动 5.1：思考时段

教师：请同学们阅读 PPT 所展示的案例，并思考如下问题，可以和同桌讨论。

问题：案例中所展示的患者/患者家属分别是基于何种理由做出了不一样的选择？

【案例 1】两位患者因心房纤颤面临脑卒中的风险。临床用于预防脑卒中的方法是服用华法林，其可使患者次年发生卒中的可能性从 2% 降至 1%。但服药后期需定期做血液检查，使活动受限，且轻度出血或大量消化道出血的风险可能增加 1%。患者 A 认为，脑卒中是一件很可怕的事，为了预防脑卒中，不在乎服用华法林、做血液检查等，即使不幸发生了消化道出血，但很快就能恢复，所以愿意选择服用华法林。患者 B 则认为，发生脑卒中虽是坏事，但尚不致命，而且发生概率低，自己平时注意的话不一定会发生。另外，自己讨厌服药，没有足够的时间定期去做血液检查，服用华法林之后出现的活动受限也会影响平时喜爱的爬山运动，服药后的消化道出血等不良反应也使人恐慌。所以不愿意服用华法林。

【案例 2】丈夫罹患前列腺癌需要进行手术，但害怕术后可能出现尿失禁、性欲减退等，因此犹豫不定甚至想放弃手术。而妻子考虑手术可让丈夫活得更长，并不在乎并发症或副作用，因此同意手术。

【案例 3】一位患者因出现严重的胸腔积液急需进行手术治疗，但其父亲却坚决拒绝手术，因为他们相信人的身体是"神圣的不可切割的"，否则整个家族都将蒙难。

（5 分钟后）

有同学愿意谈一谈以上三个案例中涉及的人物为什么会做出完全不同的选择吗？先说案例 1。

学生 1：也许是个性、生活习惯。

教师：嗯，个性、生活习惯、经历导致患者对同一治疗措施的选择完全不同。案例 2 呢？

学生 2：是对治疗效果的不同期待吧。

教师：对，是对生存质量与生存时间的考量，一个更关注生存质量、一个更则更关注生存时间。案例 3 呢？

学生 3：信仰。

教师：非常好，信仰影响了他们的选择。从上面的案例中我们看出：患者的经历、文化教育背景、宗教信仰，甚至生活状态、经济状况、婚姻、工作、亲人群体等都会影响他们对疾病的看法、对治疗方案的选择，作为医生，在进行临床决策时，一定要从患者的利益出发，充分尊重他们的价值观和愿望。那么，什么是患者的价值观呢？以下是 Gordon Guyatt 提出的定义。

患者价值观与意愿：包括患者对其健康的看法、认知、期望和目标，也包括患者对不同医疗或疾病相关选择的利弊平衡，比如潜在获益、伤害、花费及负担等。正因为存在患者的价值观与意愿这个变量，使得临床实践中，患同一疾病的患者会选择不同的治疗方案。

2. 关注患者价值观的重要性及患者的价值取向在临床诊疗决策中的限度

互动5.2：苏格拉底式提问

教师：现在我们理解了不同个体患者选择不同治疗方案的原因是他们的价值观不同，我们是否要在进行临床决策时考虑患者的价值观呢？

学生：要！

教师：当然要！但是很多时候，医生们也很难，特别是在弄清楚选择背后真正的原因之前。很多时候，患者并不会直接告诉你真实的原因。这时就需要耐心细致的工作。

在云南的一个少数民族地区，从前女性生孩子都在家里生产，导致了相当高的母婴死亡率。后来政府改进了卫生条件，新建了医院，鼓励乡民都到条件良好的医院去生产，但却发现乡民们依然选择在家中生产。为什么呢？会不会是乡村道路不好，人们到医院不方便呢？于是政府又修筑了从乡村到医院的道路，但情况依然没有改变。那是不是因为去医院生产增加了花费呢？于是政府又免去了去医院的费用，并且还增加了奖励，只要去医院生孩子都会得到一笔不少的生养费。这下大家都应该去医院生孩子了吧？可是，调查发现，大多数的家庭依然不选择去医院生产。这又是为什么呢？请大家猜一猜。

学生1：因为女人生孩子自古以来都是在家里生的，是当地人固有的价值观。

学生2：也许乡民不信任医院，害怕剖官产？

学生3：他们超生了？

学生4：也许，他们有古老的传说，认为在家里出生的孩子比较能够健康成长……

学生5：因为在妇产科里有男医生。

学生6：他们害怕医院里生孩子的人太多，婴儿可能会被抱错。

教师：很好，你们已经考虑到知识、意见、文化背景、信仰等因素可能会影响患者的选择。其实,真正的原因是当地人认为,胎盘不仅是婴儿的家,而且也是一个人一生的家,所以他们生完孩子后把胎盘埋在后院,这样当他们死后才可以回家。如果他们去医院生产,医生则一般不会把胎盘给他们。

学生 7:我明白了。完全出乎意料。

学生 8:太感人了。

教师:是的,令人感动。因此,了解患者选择背后的原因很重要,了解了原因才能找出最好的对策。而找出最好的对策也是改善医患关系、提高患者依从性的最佳方法。对于本案,大家认为最好的对策是什么?

学生 9:尊重乡民的选择,让他们在家里生孩子。

学生 10:向他们宣传科学知识,让他们放弃信仰,到医院里生孩子。

学生 11:让他们到医院里生孩子,把胎盘给他们带回去。

教师:大家觉得哪一种对策比较有效? 是的,在医院生,胎盘给他们带走。这样既可以让乡民的母婴健康得到保障,又尊重了他们的信仰和习惯,医患关系才会和谐。

学生 10:老师,我觉得向他们宣传科学知识,让他们放弃信仰,到医院里生孩子也是可行的啊。

教师:说说你怎么让人放弃自己的信仰?

学生 10:这……我不知道。

教师:我们一般很难劝人放弃自己的信仰,也是没必要的。如果信仰和治疗决策冲突,医生只有尽量解释每项医疗活动的目的、意义、风险,让患者自己做出符合自己需求的自愿选择。如果一些误解或冲突,确实是因为患者的医学知识有限而产生,医生则可以依据自己的科学训练和职业素质进行耐心解释,打消其顾虑。还有一些冲突,来自患者的经历、经验,如一位曾看着自己母亲死于乳腺癌的妇女,发现自己乳腺也有肿块时会非常惊恐。医生则不仅要运用自己的专业知识打消患者的顾虑,还应给予更多的人文关怀,以增强患者的信心,帮助患者康复。

通过以上分析,我们了解了在临床决策中,患者的价值取向是非常重要的,但是不是任何情况下都占有优先地位呢? 例如,当医生要求限制一名有较强传染性疾病患者的活动范围并对其进行隔离治疗,遭到患者拒绝时,医生是不是也要尊重他的选择呢?

学生 11:必须采取强制措施。

教师:对的,当患者自主权与社会利益发生冲突时,要优先考虑社会利益。

　　还有一种情况，患者拒绝了他不能接受的治疗方式而选择了自认为较合适的治疗方式，但该选择其实并不符合患者自己的根本利益，甚至会因拒绝治疗而丧失疾病转归的机会，从而导致死亡的可能。这种情况下，医生该如何做呢？

学生 12：尽量劝说，但尊重患者的选择。

学生 13：医生应从患者的根本利益出发，坚持自己的主张。

教师：对，医生应在合法、合情、合理的情况下坚持有利于患者根本利益的主张。这种权力，称为"医生的特殊干涉权"。

3. 决策模式

依照医生与患者在临床决策中间的角色定位，可以将决策的模式分为如下三种：患者做主模式、医生做主模式和共同决策模式。

（1）患者做主模式：患者做主模式也称单纯知照模式，是指由患者自己做出选择，医生只是提供各种方案的优点和风险等相关信息，患者根据自身的经验及理解独自做出选择。在这里患者是唯一的决策者，医生只能提供客观的信息而不掺杂个人主观成分。

（2）医生做主模式：医生做主模式也称家长作风模式，是由医生为主导，告知多少信息给患者由医生决定，医生单独或者和其他医生共同考虑收益和风险替患者做出选择，在这种情况下，患者是不参与其中的。当然这种模式是基于假定医生知道哪种方案对患者最为合适的前提下的。

（3）共同决策模式：共同决策模式（SDM）是指一种存在于医方与患方的协作关系，旨在双方共享信息、促进知情同意，确保与治疗相关的信息完全和患者共享。医学伦理学最重要的四个原则是自主原则、有利原则、不伤害原则和公正原则。医患共同决策模式是这些原则在临床应用的具体体现。是基于"以患者为中心"的临床决策，患者的自主性得到体现。共同决策模式的有效实施离不开以下几点。

A. 了解患者：医生认为最优方案与患者认为最合适自己的方案并非总是一致的。医生选择方案一般是按技术上最优来选择的，但是患者受性格、个人经历、家庭、文化与经济状况的影响，还要考虑选取某种方案后自己身体呈现的变化、对生活的影响以及费用多少等，因而并不总是按照医生的意愿和推荐进行选择。医生应当在遵循自主原则的基础上开展 SDM，了解患者对疾病的看法、对治疗的预期以及内心真正的想法，平衡技术最优与患者最合适来提供治疗方案。

如果推荐方案遭到拒绝,应当通过进一步的观察、沟通,思考被拒绝的真实原因是什么,并采取相应措施打消患者的顾虑。如果的确无法取得患者共识,则提供其他备选方案。

B. 知情同意:知情同意是 SDM 的重要步骤,只有真正让患者理解了要采取的方案、方案的风险所在、并发症以及治疗后的预期效果,才能帮助患者及其家属做出正确的选择,在出现不良事件的时候能够接受和理解。知情同意要在了解患者的基础上开展,了解他们最关注和最担心的是哪些方面。知情同意的对象理论上应该是患者本人,但现实中家属占据重要地位,因而最好的方式应该是两方共同参与,如果双方意见不一,需要医生从中协调。

C. 选择方案:医生在 SDM 中的角色是提供专业意见,帮助患者做出决定。医生首先从专业最优的角度做出初步选择,然后根据患者的心理与社会因素(包括性别、年龄、家庭角色、工作、对治疗的预期等)进行考虑,在风险与受益、长期与短期效果、发展新技术与患者的安全、性与价等之间取得平衡。例如,在不得不选择截肢术的时候,对患者及家属的劝说应强调延误治疗的严重后果、目前先进的假肢技术在帮助患者恢复功能、重返生活方面的效果。如果患者需要维持较好的运动功能,则建议患者选择关节置换。考虑患者的支付能力,如果患者经济困难,则选择尽管疗效不是最佳但是性价比高的替代方案。

4. 决策辅助系统

循证医学的理念要求基于现有最好的证据,兼顾医生的临床经验以及患者的价值观和意愿,进行医学实践。尽管当前各种临床指南已指出患者应和医生共同决策,以确定最终的诊疗方案。然而在实际临床实践中,患者的参与程度并不高,而且经常会因为缺乏相关医学知识而陷入选择矛盾中,无法真正地参与医疗决策。因此,向患者提供基于循证医学证据的、与治疗方案选择相关的信息十分必要。

患者决策辅助系统是帮助患者参与临床决策过程的一种工具。它以证据为基础,帮助患者详细了解不同治疗方案的益处和风险,平衡患者的综合需求。患者决策辅助系统的适用范围很广,如是否进行疾病筛查或诊断试验、选择保守治疗或手术治疗、是否改变不良的生活方式等。除成年疾病外,此工具也可应用于儿童健康的某些领域。它充分体现了“患者自我管理”的观念,受到患者和临床医生的认可。

成立于 2003 年的国际患者决策辅助标准(IPDAS)协作组织,其主要任务是建立统一的质量评价体系,加强患者决策辅助系统的质量和效果管理。该组织为患者决策辅助系统的内容、发展、使用和评估提供了一整套基于循证医学的框架体系。

患者决策辅助系统的形式包括宣传手册、录音带、视频或互动网页等。与传统的健康宣传材料相比,患者决策辅助系统强调治疗方案的多样性,详细描述了各种方案的风险和益处并明确表明各自的发生概率,其内容更具针对性。此外,一些患者决策辅助体系提供了价值观及偏好阐明训练,帮助患者及医生了解真正的治疗需求。患者可以在临床咨询前或咨询时使用,明确自己对不同治疗方式的偏好,针对性地进行咨询,提高其决策满意度。

5. 共同决策模式实践

互动5.3: 门诊角色扮演

教师: 请同学先阅读并熟悉以下案例,明确不同角色的身份和处境。所有同学自由组合,以三人为一小组,每小组内有一位同学扮演孕妇,一位同学扮演丈夫,一位扮演医生,模拟决策的过程。希望同学们运用前面学习的内容,让这对母婴有不一样的结局。你们有10分钟的准备时间,然后我将请同学们上来表演。

【案例】 一产妇,身材娇小,骨盆狭窄,临产时经试产无法顺利分娩,医生决定采用剖宫产,于是将产妇情况告诉产妇丈夫。但其丈夫却拖延不签字。其拒签的理由并不是担心妻子接受剖宫产有风险,而是顾虑妻子这次生的是女儿,会因剖宫产影响下次男孩的生产。产妇再三请求医生为其实施剖宫产。而医生以家属没有签字为理由没有及时做手术。结果导致产妇子宫破裂,此时才进手术室实施子宫全切术,但为时已晚,母婴俱亡。

教师: 哪一个组先来表演?
学生: (分别进行角色扮演)

李红梅   刘   敏

Chapter 5

Patients' Values in Clinical Practice

Part I Teaching Requirements

EBM emphasizes the combination of the best evidences, doctors' expertise and patients' values. Therefore, how to effectively incorporate patients' values and preferences into personalized clinical decision-making, will be an important challenge confronting the development of EBM. It is hoped that, by studing this chapter, students can master the definition, differences and limits of patients' values, so as to be familiar with common patient decision aids and shared decision model (SDM) in decision-making patterns; and to learn how to guide the patient' values correctly in practice.

1. Teaching aims

Master the definition and meaning of patients' values and preferences, and be able to use patient decision aids and the shared decision model to help patients play a part in exploring the causes as well as in treatment planning.

2. Leaning objectives

After completing this session, students should be able to:

(1) Describe the definition of patients' values and preferences, differences and limitations of patients' values and preferences in clinical decision-making.

(2) Describe the commonly-used patient decision aids and shared decision model (SDM).

(3) Choose appropriate methods to guide the patients' values in practice.

3. Teaching methods

This session will use lecture，PPT presentation and interactive teaching method. Interactive teaching techniques include think break，socratic questioning and out-patient role-play.

4. Reading materials

（1）Alonso-Coello P，Montori V M，Díaz M G，et al. Values and preferences for oral antithrombotic therapy in patients with atrial fibrillation：physician and patient perspectives. Health Expect.，2015，18(6)：2318 - 2327.

（2）Maclean S，Mulla S，Akl E A，et al. Patient values and preferences in decision making for antithrombotic therapy：a systematic review：antithrombotic therapy and prevention of thrombosis，9th ed：American college of chest physicians evidence-based clinical practice guidelines. Chest，2012，141(2)：e1S - 23S.

Part II　Teaching Design — 2 periods（80 minutes）

Teaching design of "Patients' Values in Clinical Practice"

No.	Content	Interactive technique/ teaching techniques	Descriptions	Time (minutes)
1	Definition of patients' values and differences	PPT presentation Interaction 5.1: Think break	Show students the cases on PPT, let them think and discuss with their deskmates, and then introduce the definition proposed by Gordon Guyatt.	10
2	The importance and limitations of patients' values	Interaction 5.2: Socratic questioning	Through a series of questions, the teacher draws out the differences of patients' values, its importance and limitations in clinical diagnosis and treatment decisions-making.	30
3	Clinical decision-making model	PPT presentation	Clinical decision model and the keys of shared decision model.	15
4	Patient decision aids	PPT presentation	Help patients understand the benefits and risks of different treatments and balance their expectations based on evidence.	5

（continued）

No.	Content	Interactive technique/ teaching techniques	Descriptions	Time (minutes)
5	Shared decision model (SDM).	Interaction 5.3: Out-patient role-play	Through out-patient role-play, students can understand the work of patients' values in clinical decision-making and get familiar with the shared decision model.	20

Part III   Teaching Contents

1. Definition of the patients' values

Interaction 5.1 : Think break

Teacher: Please read the case presented in PPT and think about the following question. You may discuss with your deskmates. For what reasons did the patients/family members shown in the case make different choices?

[Case 1] Two patients with atrial fibrillation are faced with the risk of stroke. If taking warfarin, the possibility of stroke in the next year will decline down from 2% to 1%. But a regular blood test should be done at the later stage, activities may be limited, and the risk of mild bleeding or massive gastrointestinal bleeding may increase by 1%. According to Patient A, stroke is a very terrible thing. In order to prevent stroke, he does not care about taking warfarin or doing blood tests. Even if the gastrointestinal bleeding happens unfortunately, it may recover quickly, so he would like to take warfarin, while patient B believes that stroke is severe but not fatal, and the probability of occurrence is low. If he is cautious enough, it may not have to happen. In addition, He hates to take drugs, and there is no enough time for him to do regular blood tests. Activity restrictions after taking warfarin will also affect the usual favorite mountain climbing, and gastrointestinal bleeding after medication and other adverse effects also make him panic. So eventually he would not like to take warfarin.

【Case 2】The husband suffers from prostate cancer and needs a surgery, but is afraid of the possibility of urinary incontinence, loss of libido, etc.. So he hesitates and even wants to give up the operation, while the wife considers that the surgery will keep the husband alive longer, and she doesn't care about the complications or side effects, so agrees with the surgery.

【Case 3】A patient is in urgent need of surgery because of severe hydrothorax, but his father refuses the operation because they believes that the human body is "sacred and non-cutting". Otherwise the whole family will be in trouble.

（5 minutes later）

Would anybody like to talk about why the characters involved in the above three cases make completely different choices? Let's start with case 1.

Students 1: Maybe it's personality and living habits.

Teacher: Well, personality, lifestyle, experience lead to a completely different choice of one treatment. What about case 2?

Student 2: It's different depending on expectations to treatment effects.

Teacher: Yes, it's a trade-off between quality of life and survival time. One pays more attention to quality of life and the other pays more attention to survival time. What about case 3?

Student 3: Faith.

Teacher: Very good, the faith affected their choices. We can see from the above cases, the patient experiences, cultural background, religious belief, education and living conditions, economy, marriage, work, family group will influence their perceptions of diseases, such as choice of treatments. As a doctor, when making clinical decisions, he must be in the interests of the patients, fully respect their values and aspirations. So what is patients' values? The following is the definition proposed by Gordon Guyatt.

Patients' values and preferences: Gordon Guyatt thinks that Patients' values and preferences include patients' perceptions, expectations and goals of their health, as well as patients' balance of advantages and disadvantages of different medical or disease-related choices, such as potential benefits, harms, costs and burdens. Because of the variable value and willingness of patients, patients with the same disease will choose different treatment options in clinical practice.

2. Importance and limitations of patients' values in clinical diagnosis and treatment decisions

Interaction 5.2 : Socratic questioning

Teacher: Now, we understand the reason why different individual patient chooses different treatment option is that they have different values. Should we consider patients' values when making clinical decisions?

Class: Yes!

Teacher: Yes, of course! But sometimes it is very different to deal with them before we know the deeper original reasons. Sometimes, patients may not tell you the real reason directly. Therefore we need more patience. In an ethnic group region of Yunnan province in China, women used to give birth at home, leading to high maternal and infant mortality rates. Later, the government improved the sanitary conditions and built a new hospital, encouraging the villagers to give birth in the well-conditioned hospital. But the villagers still chose to give birth at home. Why? Could it be that the country roads were so bad that people couldn't get to the hospital? So the government built roads from the countryside to the hospital, but nothing changed. Well, was it because of the increased cost of going to the hospital? So the government waived the cost of giving birth in hospital, and also increased the reward. Whoever gives birth in the hospital will get a lot of birth subsidies. Now, would people go to the hospital to give birth? However, the survey found that most families still did not choose to go to the hospital to give birth. Why is that? Please have a guess.

Student 1: Because women have been giving birth at home since ancient times, which is the inherent value of local people.

Student 2：Maybe villagers didn't believe the hospital，for fear of caesarean?

Student 3：They had broken "one child" policy before?

Student 4：Maybe there was an old local saying that children born at home would grow up more healthily ...

Student 5：Because there were male doctors in obstetrics and gynecology department.

Student 6：Be afraid of so many people giving birth at the hospital that the babies might be taken wrongly.

Teacher：Very good，you have already considered the fact that knowledge，opinion，cultural background，belief and other reasons may affect the choice of the patients. Actually the real reason is that the local people believe the placenta is not only a baby's home but also a lifelong home，so they bury the placenta in their backyard after giving birth so that they can go home after death. And if they go to the hospital to give birth，doctors won't give them the placenta.

Student 7：I see. Totally unexpected.

Student 8：It's so moving.

Teacher：Yes，it is moving. Therefore，it is important to understand the reasons behind patients' selections and find out the best solutions. It is also the best way to improve the doctor-patient relationship and patients' compliance. What do you think is the best solution to this case?

Student 9：Respect the choices of the villagers and let them give birth at home.

Student 10：Educate them，and let them give up the faith and give birth in the hospital.

students 11：Ask them to give birth in the hospital and let them take back the placenta.

Teacher：What do you think? What kind of approach is more effective? Yes，giving birth in the hospital and taking back the placenta with them. It can not only guarantee the maternal and infant health of the villagers，but also respect their beliefs and habits，so that the doctor-patient relationship can be harmonious.

Student 10: Teacher, I think it is feasible to spread scientific knowledge to them and make them give up their beliefs.

Teacher: Ok, could you tell me about how you will let the people give up their beliefs?

Student 10: This ... I don't know.

Teacher: Generally, it is difficult to convince people to give up their beliefs. Actually it's not necessary. If beliefs and treatment decisions conflict, what a doctor can do is trying to explain the purpose, meaningfulness, and the risk of each medical activity, and then allow the patients to make their own choices that meet their needs. If some misunderstandings or conflicts are indeed caused by patients' limitation of medical knowledge, doctors must explain to them patiently according to their scientific trainings, professional qualities and dispel their concerns. Other conflicts come from the patient's past experiences. A woman who watched her mother died of breast cancer and was horrified to find a lump in her breast. Doctors should not only use their professional knowledge to dispel the patient's concerns, but also give more humanistic care to enhance the patient's confidence and help her recover.

Through the above analyses, we know in clinical decision-making, the value orientation of patients is very important, but whether the value orientation in all cases has the priority or not? For example, should a doctor also need to respect the patient's choice of declining isolation method when this patient is with a highly contagious disease.

Student 11: Compulsory measures must be taken.

Teacher: Right, when a patient's autonomy conflicts with social interests, social interests should be prioritized.

Another situation is that the patient chooses the treatment that he or she thinks is more suitable while rejecting the treatment that he or she cannot accept. However, the choice is actually not in his or her fundamental interests. They may even lose the chance of recovery due to refusing treatment, leading to death. What should a doctor do in this situation?

Student 12: Try to persuade, but respect the patient's choice.

Student 13: Doctors should first consider the fundamental interests of patients and stick to their own opinions.

Teacher: Yes, doctors should adhere to the proposition that is beneficial to the fundamental interests of patients under the legal and reasonable conditions. This right is called "the doctor's special right of intervention".

3. Decision model

According to the role of doctors and patients playing in clinical decision-making, the model of decision-making can be divided into the following three types: patients' decision model, doctors' decision model and shared decision model (SDM).

(1) Patients' decision model: It is also called the pure informed model, which refers to patients making a choice by themselves. The doctor just provides information about the advantages and risks of various options, and the patients make the choice by themselves according to the experience and understanding alone. Patients are the only decision-makers here, and doctors can only provide objective information without involving personal subjectivity.

(2) Doctors' decision model: It is also called the paternalistic model. Decision-making is dominated by doctors. That how much information should be given to the patients is determined by the doctor. The doctor alone, or together with other doctors, makes a choice after considering the benefits and risks for the patients. In this case, the patient is not involved. This model, of course, is based on the assumption that the doctor knows which option is the best one for the patient.

(3) Shared decision model (SDM): It refers to a collaborative relationship between doctors and patients, which aims to share information, promote informed consent, and ensure that the information related to treatment is fully shared with patients. The most important four principles of medical ethics are autonomous principle, benefit principle, no harm principle

and fair principle. The shared decision model is the concrete embodiment of these principles in clinical application. This model is based on the "patient-centered" clinical decision, in which the patient's autonomy is reflected.

Effective implementation of the shared decision model is inseparable from the following aspects:

A. To understand your patients: The optimal solution in doctors' mind is not always consistent with the patient's choice. Doctors generally consider more of whether the treatment is technically optimal, but the choice of a patient is affected not only by personality, personal experience, the influence of family, cultural and economic conditions, but also by the changes of his/her body after selecting a program, the impact on the life, the cost and so on. Therefore patients don't always make decisions according to the doctor's will and recommendations. Doctors should carry out SDM on the basis of following the principles of autonomy, understanding patients' views on the disease, their expectations on treatment and inner real thoughts, so that the doctors can balance the optimal technology and the most appropriate treatments to patients. If the recommended solution is rejected, the true reason for the rejection should be considered through further observation and communication, and relevant measures should be taken to dispel patients' concerns. If consensus cannot be reached, alternative options should be provided.

B. Informed consent: Informed consent is an important step of SDM. Only when the patient truly understands the plan to be adopted and the risk of the plan, complications and expected effects, can the patient and his family be helped to make right choices and be able to accept and understand when adverse events occur. Informed consent should be carried out on the basis of understanding the patients and what they are most concerned about. In theory, the object of informed consent should be the patient himself, but in reality, family members also take an important position, so the best way should be the joint participation of both parties. If the two parties disagree, doctors should coordinate between them.

C. To select options: The role of doctors playing in SDM is to provide professional advice to help patients make decisions. Doctors firstly make a preliminary selection from professional perspective, and then take the patient's psychological and social factors（including gender，age，family roles，work，and expectations of treatment，etc.）into account，and balance the risks and benefits，long-term and short-term effects，development of new technology and the patient's safety. For example，at the time of the choice of amputation，the persuasion to the patients and their families should be focused on the serious consequences of the delay，and the fact that the present advanced prosthetic techniques can help restore the function and help the patients return to life. If patients need to maintain better motor function，it is suggested that patients should choose replacement. Considering the patient's ability to pay，if the patient is in financial difficulties，choose an alternative that is not optimal but cost-effective despite the fact that the effect is not optimal.

4. Decision support system

The concept of EBM requires both medical practice based on the best available evidence，and taking the doctor's clinical experience and the patient's values and preferences into account. Although，by the current clinical guidelines，it has been pointed out that patients should make decisions together with doctors to determine the final diagnosis and treatment plan；however，in actual clinical practice，patients are not involved in a high degree of participation and often fall into a conflict of choice due to the lack of relevant medical knowledge and they can't really participate in medical decisions. So it is very necessary to provide patients with information based on EBM and treatment options.

Patient decision aids system is a tool to help patients participate in clinical decision-making process. It helps patients understand the benefits and risks of different treatments and balance the patients' needs based on evidence. The patient decision support system has a wide range of applications，such as whether to carry out the disease screening，diagnosis test，select conservative treatment，surgical treatment，change unhealthy lifestyles or not. In addition to adult diseases，this tool can also be applied in certain areas of children's health. It fully embodies the concept of "patient self-management" and has been recognized by patients and clinicians.

The collaborative organization of the International Patient Decision

Aided Standards (IPDAS) was established in 2003. Its main task is to establish a unified quality assessment system and strengthen the quality and effectiveness of patient decision support systems. The organization provides a complete framework based on EBM with the content, development, use, and evaluation of patient decision support systems.

The form of patient decision support system includes brochures, audiotapes, videos or interactive web pages. Compared with the traditional health publicity materials, the patient decision support system emphasizes the diversity of the treatment scheme, describes the risks and benefits of various schemes in detail, and clearly indicates the probability of their respective occurrence. Its contents are more targeted. In addition, some patient decision support systems provide values and preferences clarification training to help patients and doctors understand the true need for treatment. Patients can use it before or during clinical consultations to clarify their own preferences for different treatment methods, and conduct targeted consultation to improve their satisfaction with decision-making.

5. Practice of shared decision model

Interaction 5.3 : Out-patient role-play

Teacher: Please read and familiarize yourself with the following case. Clarify and remember the identities and situations of different roles. All of you come together freely, in groups of three. In each group, one student acts as a pregnant woman, one as a husband and one as a doctor, simulating the decision-making process. I hope you can use what you've learnt previously, so that this mother and baby have a different outcome. You have 10 minutes to prepare, and then I'm going to select some of you to come up and perform in public.

【Case】 A lying-in woman, petite, with contracted pelvis, could not give natural birth after the trial of labor, the doctor decided to adopt a caesarean section, so informed the husband of the condition. But her husband delayed and avoided signature. The reason for his refusal was not that he was worried about the risks of a cesarean section his wife was going to take, but that she was giving birth to a daughter, and the cesarean delivery could affect the next boy's birth. The mother repeatedly asked the doctor for a cesarean. The doctor did not perform the operation in time on the ground that the family did not sign it. The result was a rupture of the uterus. At this time, a total hysterectomy was performed in the operating room, but it was too late and both mother and baby died.

Teacher: Which group is going to perform firstly?

Students: (to role-play respectively)

Li Hongmei　Liu Min

第6章

治疗性研究的严格评价

第一部分　教　学　要　求

该环节主要是关于如何严格地评价治疗性研究证据。目的在于帮助学生了解医学干预性研究文献的真实性、重要性和相关性,能够独立地对文献报道的信息进行解读和判断。学生将了解到对文献的严格评价是实践循证医学的基础。

1. 教学目的

介绍如何应用循证技术构建可回答的治疗性问题,检索文献并严格地评价文献,从而有效鉴别医疗干预措施。

2. 学习目标

通过此环节的学习,学生能够:

(1) 构建可回答的治疗性问题。

(2) 描述治疗性研究评价的三个方面(真实性、重要性和相关性)。

(3) 列出影响 RCT 真实性的偏倚类型。

(4) 理解临床显著性的意义、可信区间、治疗效果的测量指标和效应量(OR/RR)。

(5) 根据试验报告的结果计算 RR、NNT。

(6) 理解把研究结果应用到当前患者时要考虑的问题。

3. 教学方法

此环节采用讲授法、PPT 演示和互动教学法,互动教学技术包括 TPR、教师讲故事和 TPS。

4. 阅读材料

(1) Beausoleil M. Effect of a fermented milk combining *Lactobacillus*

acidophilus Cl1285 and *Lactobacillus casei* in the prevention of antibiotic-associated diarrhea：a randomized，double-blind，placebo-controlled trial. Can J Gastroenterol，2007，21(11)：732-736.

(2) Guyatt G H，Sackett D L，Cook D J，et al. Users' guides to the medical literature：II. How to use an article about therapy or prevention：A. Are the results of the study valid?. Jama，1993，270(21)：2598-2601.

第二部分　教学设计——2 课时（80 分钟）

"治疗性研究的严格评价"教学设计表

序号	内　容	互动技术/教学技术	描　　　述	时间（分钟）
1	复习	互动 6.1：TPR	采用 TPR 技术回顾上周所学	10
2	真实性评价	PPT 演示	介绍以下内容：治疗与治疗性问题的概念；治疗性问题的最佳证据；影响治疗性研究结果的因素及对策	15
3	一个临床故事	互动 6.2：教师讲故事	教师描述一个真实的故事，询问学生如何遵循循证医学的原则解决相关问题	10
4	真实性评价实践	互动 6.3：TPS	介绍真实性评价工作表（见附录Ⅳ），让学生阅读 Beausoleil M 的文献并填写工作表，讨论并与全班分享	15
5	重要性评价	PPT 演示	介绍治疗性研究的重要性评价内容，着重介绍治疗性研究的效应量计算方法、准确性和可信区间	15
6	重要性评价实践	互动 6.4：TPS	学生完成基于 Beausoleil M 研究的计算任务	10
7	相关性评价	PPT 演示	介绍应用证据前应考虑的诸多方面，提醒学生完成工作表 3 及 KWL 表	5

第三部分 教 学 内 容

1. 复习：采用 TPR 技术回顾上周所学

互动 6.1： TPR

教师：各位早上好！让我们从你们的 KWL 表开始。请快速浏览一下你们的 KWL 表。两分钟后，我会就你们之前学过的内容提问。如果你认为描述是正确的，请站起来，如果你认为描述是错误的，请继续坐着。

现在，各位准备好了吗？

(1) 循证医学的三个基本要素是证据、医生和医疗设施。正确或错误？

学生：（反馈）

教师：(2) 证据分类和分组的重要依据之一是流行病学的研究设计。正确或错误？

学生：（反馈）

教师：(3) 第一个提出"循证医学"定义的学者是 Archie Cochrane。正确或错误？

学生：（反馈）

教师：(4) 构建一个基于证据的临床问题，你不需要考虑结局。正确或错误？

学生：（反馈）

教师：(5) 构建一个基于证据的临床问题，你需要考虑 PICO。正确或错误？

学生：（反馈）

教师：(6) 循证医学基于最好的证据、医生的医学素养及患者的价值观。正确或错误？

学生：（反馈）

教师：(7) 6S 模型将证据资源分为六类：系统、总结、摘要、合成、原始研究的合成及原始研究。正确或错误？

学生：（反馈）

教师：(8) 根据循证医学实践的 5As，检索证据是循证实践的第二个步骤。正确或错误？

学生：（反馈）

> **教师**：（9）证据分类和分级的目的是更有效地利用证据。正确或错误？
> **学生**：（反馈）
> **教师**：（10）证据的分类和分是基于研究设计的不同。正确或错误？
> **学生**：（反馈）
> **教师**：（11）证据金字塔是一个 8 级系统，第一次将动物实验和体外研纳入证据体系。正确或错误？
> **学生**：（反馈）
> **教师**：（12）可以将证据分为两大类：原始研究证据和二次研究证据。正确或错误？
> **学生**：（反馈）

2. 概述

从某种意义上说，临床实践是一个回答一系列问题并做出临床决策的过程。循证医学实践强调运用当前可获得的最佳证据进行临床决策。而最好的证据通常来自设计、实施完好的患者为导向的研究（poems 研究）。来自良好研究的结果能够反映实验对象的真实情况（即具有内部真实性），同时其研究结果能够推断整体真值（即具有外部真实性）。今天我们将要学习如何鉴别一个好的治疗性研究。

（1）"治疗"的参考范畴和"治疗性问题"：治疗通常是指针对健康问题进行尝试性修复的过程，常常在诊断后实施。在医疗领域，therapy 与 treatment 两者意思相同。其他一些英文表达如 care、intervention、therapy 和 treatment，彼此语义重叠，结合上下文可以作为同义词使用。治疗主要是指对个体的干预，如药物疗法、手术疗法、康复、护理、心理疗法、改变生活方式（如戒烟、运动疗法、饮食疗法），有时也指对社会群体的干预（如健康教育计划、阅读疗法、群体干预、预防和控制、疾病筛查）。

治疗性问题是指关于干预的有效性和安全性问题。在所有临床问题中，治疗性问题占了很大的比例。临床任务是解决如何选择治疗方法，即向患者提供利大于弊、经济而有效的治疗方法。治疗性研究旨在回答治疗性问题。

（2）治疗性问题的最佳证据：回答治疗性问题的最好证据是什么呢？请回忆我们曾经学过的证据金字塔（见第 3 章）。在这个等级结构中，不同的研究或信息源能提供不同级别的证据，证据的级别是基于不同的研究设计的。因此，对治疗性问题，一般来说，系统评价、荟萃分析和大型随机对照试验的结果可认为是治疗的金标准。然而,无论系统评价或临床研究的类型和来源如何,所有的证据都需要经过严格评价。例如,一个具有确定结果,以及基于同质性原始研究基础上的高质量的系统评价代表最高水平的证据。大型的、有确定结果的随机对照试验(可信区间不包含无效值)相对不确定结果的随机对照试验(点估计值有临床显著性但可信区间包含无效值)而言,是更好的证据。一个精心设计的大型队列研究有可能提供比方法上有严重缺陷的随机对照研究更有效的证据。

(3) 影响治疗性研究结果的因素与对策

A. 机遇与偏倚:机遇是指由概率造成的测量值(观察值)与真实值的差异,可导致随机误差。其大小可以用统计学方法进行估计,但没有方向性,即这种误差表现为测量值随机地高于或低于真值。随机误差在抽样研究时不可避免,我们只能将其控制在一定的范围内。偏倚即系统误差,是指由于研究人员、设备或研究方法等因素导致观察值与真实值之间的偏离。与机遇不同,偏倚的存在总是造成研究结果高于或低于真实值,因而是有方向性的。在研究工作中很难定量估计偏倚的大小,而研究偏倚方向则相对比较容易。在研究过程中,会产生各种不同类型的偏倚,如选择性偏倚、测量偏倚、混杂偏倚等,主要通过严格的设计加以避免,随机分配能最大限度地避免选择性偏倚。

B. 样本量:样本量的大小直接反映受机遇影响的程度。小样本研究容易受机遇的影响,出现假阳性和假阴性的可能性比较大。样本量越大,受机遇影响越小,研究结果越接近于真实。

C. 依从性:是指研究对象按研究要求执行医嘱的客观应答程度。在新药临床试验中,依从性可定义为受试者按照规定的药物剂量和疗程服用试验药物的程度。受试者的依从性与试验结果的质量密不可分,不依从或依从性差是导致治疗无效的最常见原因,在新药临床试验中不依从的情况非常普遍。据统计,完全依从、依从性差和完全不依从的受试者约各占 1/3。提高依从性的措施包括:加强患者依从性教育,尽量选择简单、易行的治疗方案,改善医务人员的服务态度和医疗技术水平,及时处理药物不良反应等。

D. 向均数回归现象:是指某些具有异常测量指标的患者即使不接受治疗,在其后的连续测量中,这些指标也有向正常值接近的趋势。这种现象可能因测量值围绕均值上下波动引起,也可能是测量指标的生理波动,而非干预所致。向均数回归现象可以造成治疗有效的假象。对同一个体的相关测量指标,在相同条件下,不同时间多次测量后取其均值,可以减少其对结果的影响。

E. 沾染和干扰:沾染是指对照组研究对象有意或无意接受了试验组的治疗。沾染会使试验组和对照组之间可能存在的差异减少。干扰是指试验组或对照组的研究对象额外接受了类似试验措施的其他处理,从而人为地影响试验措施的疗效。沾染和干扰可以通过双盲或三盲设计加以避免。

F. 霍桑效应：是指研究过程中研究者可能对自己感兴趣的对象关注更多，当研究对象成为被关注的目标时往往有意或无意地改善自我行为，从而夸大治疗效果。避免霍桑效应的方法是设立对照组，并采用双盲或三盲设计。

3. 临床案例

互动 6.2：教师讲故事

教师讲述一个真实的故事或经历，启发学生思考如何应用循证医学的原理解决问题。

教师：我要告诉你们一个真实的故事。我朋友的母亲，今年 70 岁了，但仍然很有活力。最近她不幸在家中跌倒，被送至急诊室，行医学检查后发现右股骨骨折。医生建议马上进行手术并且术前给予抗生素。朋友来咨询我的意见。因为我曾经读到过一些关于老年人抗生素相关性腹泻的文章，所以我请她问问医生，是否可以在使用抗生素时服用一些含乳酸菌的酸奶或其他益生菌类产品以预防可能出现的抗生素相关性腹泻。但医生没有提供明确的答案。如果我想自己亲自实践一下循证医学来寻找答案，我应该怎么做呢？你们能告诉我实践循证医学的步骤吗？

学生 1：提出问题，查到证据，评价证据，应用证据，后效评价。

教师：太棒了！首先，让我们从第一步开始，提出临床问题，我这里有三个问题，你们认为哪一个是最好的临床问题？

A：什么方法治疗腹泻最好？

B：服用抗生素的患者，同时服用益生菌能预防腹泻吗？

C：益生菌能预防老年住院患者抗生素相关性腹泻吗？

学生 2：C。

教师：非常好！现在我们进行第二步。以下是三个检索策略，如果我们选择 PubMed 数据库，哪一个最能检索到关于这个临床问题的证据？

A：diarrhea AND best treatment Limited to free full text.

B：diarrhea AND probiotics AND elderly AND female AND adult Limited to English.

C：antibiotics AND diarrhea AND probioticsLimited to Meta-analysis，systematic review，randomized controlled trial.

学生 3：C。

教师： 很好！我们采用 C 策略在 PubMed 中检索，可以检索到很多研究证据包括荟萃分析、系统评价、随机对照试验等。好，再让我们来实践循证医学第三个步骤——证据的评价。如何来评价一个治疗性研究证据呢？我将发给大家这个评价工作表。

4. 真实性评价任务

向学生介绍真实性严格评价工作表。请学生阅读 Beausoleil M 的文献，自己完成工作表，与同桌讨论并与全班分享。

互动 6.3：TPS

教师： 通过对临床问题的检索，我们获得检索结果，在这些结果中包括有最高级别的临床证据如 SR 和 Meta 分析，也有许多原始研究。在应用这些证据帮助我们进行临床决策之前，必须先对证据进行评价。对于 SR 和 Meta 分析的评价，我们将于后面的章节讨论。今天我们将着重于如何评价原始研究证据。Beausoleil M 的文献是一篇原始研究。文章所报道的研究结果真实吗？请大家阅读这篇文献并完成工作表 1，工作表 1 是用于真实性严格评价的工作表。大家可以和同桌讨论，然后我会请各位来与全班同学分享你的答案。大家有 15 分钟完成这项任务。

工作表 1：治疗性研究的真实性评价

此研究的结果是否真实？	是	否	不清楚
1. 研究对象（患者）的分组随机吗？			
2. 分配方案是隐匿的吗？			
3. 试验开始时各组基线可比吗？			
4. 对患者、医生和研究者是否采用了盲法？			
5. 随访完整吗？随访时长是否足够？			
6. 患者是否恰当地归入所属分组进行分析计算？			
7. 各组除了试验的治疗措施不同外，其他医疗措施都相同吗？			

学生： （阅读和讨论）

教师： 时间到，让我们看看你们的答案。

第 1 条,"患者是随机分组的吗?"是的！该文报道了患者是随机分配的。但是它并没有详细描述是如何随机的。因此难以判断研究是不是真正的随机分组。那么什么是随机? 为什么随机如此重要呢?

学生：随机化是随机抽样,是为了减少偏倚。

教师：对。随机化是临床科学研究的重要方法和基本原则,包括受试者被随机抽样并随机分配到干预组和对照组。选择性偏倚源于各组间的某种特征上的差异,使组间缺乏可比性。采用恰当的方法(如计算机产生的随机数字),将研究对象随机分配到对照组和实验组可以消除潜在的偏倚。采用交替分组或医院就诊号/住院号分配方案时,调查者也有可能破坏随机方案,此外,不充分的分配隐藏也是一个偏倚的重要来源,因此调查者应保持无法知晓分配方案。

现在,我们来看第 2 条,"分配是否隐藏?"是或否? 不清楚。文章并没有提供足够的信息帮助我们判断是否进行了分配隐藏。为什么分配隐藏很重要呢?

学生：防止研究者破坏随机过程。

教师：正确,我们在第 1 条里讨论过了。

第 3 条,基线特征,是否所有影响预后的指标在组间一致? 是的,文献中表 1 显示了基线特征。值得注意的是实验中安慰剂组服用 laxatives 和 beta-lactams 的人数较多。同学们可以思考一下,这个差异是否会影响试验结果。我们为什么要考查基线水平?

学生：为了保持组间的平衡和可比性。

教师：很好！第 4 条,是否采用盲法? 是的,患者采用了盲法。为两组患者提供的药品看起来都一样,品味和质地也是相同的。然而,虽然文中提到这是一个双盲试验,但未清楚表明另外一个盲法对象是谁。为什么盲法如此重要?

学生：为了减少来自研究者或研究对象的主观影响。

教师：对的,如霍桑效应,还有呢? 盲法还可减少执行偏倚和测量偏倚。

执行偏倚源于受试者和研究执行人员对所分配的干预措施的理解差异。双盲法常常用于预防此类偏倚,因为此时无论受试者或是研究人员都不知道受试者被施加的干预措施是什么。双盲法也可防止对安慰剂作用的抵触,尤其是对于测量结局为一些主观指标,如疼痛的研究来说是非常重要的。当对两组结局指标的测量或评估方法不同时,测量偏倚就会产生。如果可能的话,应对结局的评估应采用盲法。

第 5 条,随访。随访完整吗? 时间足够长吗? 此文中是否提供了相关证据?

学生:随访是完整的。他们提供了所有研究对象最后一次抗生素给药后 21 天的随访信息。

教师:理想状态下,所有研究对象均应完成试验并取得相关数据。如果接受试验治疗的患者因为副作用而退出试验,他们的数据不参与数据分析,这样会高估试验疗法的疗效。一般来说,失访率应控制在 10% 以内,特殊情况下失访率也不能超过 20%。另外,我们还应确保随访时间足够以观察到临床效果。

第 6 条,患者是否恰当地归入所属分组进行分析计算? 即是否遵循意向性治疗分析原则? 是的,该研究报道了一级和二级结局指标均基于意向性治疗原则进行分析。但是,什么是意向性治疗分析呢?

意向性治疗分析是指不论受试者是否接受了最初分配的治疗方案(包括中途停药或接受了其他治疗),均应按照原来的分组进行统计分析。观察研究证实,对于中途退出的受试对象来说,治疗效果通常都会比完成试验的受试对象差,因此,分析中不纳入这些受试对象,则会导致高估治疗的效果。意向性治疗分析主要用于防止失访偏倚,是由于参与者退出研究,或由于违反协议,使组间出现的系统性差异。

第 7 条,除试验措施外,组间接受的其他处理是否一致?

学生:是的。

教师:为什么我们需要均等治疗?

学生:保持组间平衡。

教师:对,防止混杂偏倚。混杂是由于存在外在的一种或多种因素,使暴露因素和结局之间的关系受到混淆或干扰。到此,我们已经完成了治疗性研究的真实性评价。请按刚才我们谈到的及下表所示修正你们的真实性评价表。记住真实性评价的 7 个方面。下面我们将要学习重要性评价的内容。

工作表 1: 治疗性研究的真实性评价(核对)

此研究的结果是否真实?	是	否	不清楚
1.患者的分组随机吗?	√		
2.随机化过程是隐匿的吗?			√
3.试验开始时各组情况相似吗?	√		

（续表）

此研究的结果是否真实？	是	否	不清楚
4. 对患者、医生和研究者是否采用了盲法？	√		
5. 随访完整吗？随访时长是否足够？	√		
6. 患者是否恰当地归入所属分组进行分析计算？	√		
7. 各组除了试验的治疗措施不同外，其它医疗措施都相同吗？	√		

5. 重要性评价（研究结果是什么？结果的准确性如何？是否能改变我的临床决策？）

证据的重要性评价应在确定真实性的基础上进行。重要性评价包括评估治疗的效应量和精确度。

（1）治疗效果的测量：循证医学评估治疗效果的大小常用两类统计学指标，一类用于分析计数资料（如疾病的发生率、病死率等），另一类用于分析计量资料（如血压、血糖、身高、体重等）。

A. 分析计数资料的常用统计学指标：假设一个平行随机安慰剂对照试验，随访时间足够长，研究目的是预防一种不良事件（如死亡），治疗的效果反映为两种结局（事件发生/事件不发生），则可计算以下指标。

- 对照组的事件发生率（CER）：CER=对照组某事件的发生率。
- 试验组的事件发生率（EER）：EER=试验组某事件的发生率。
- 绝对危险度降低率（ARR）：对照组和试验组不良结局事件发生率的差值，ARR=CER−EER。
- 相对危险度（RR）：试验组事件发生率与对照组事件发生率的比值，RR=EER/CER，RR=1 表示空值或无差别。
- 相对危险度降低率（RRR）：与相对危险度有关，可以通过以下公式计算，RRR=1−RR。相对危险度降低率可反映试验组与对照组事件发生率降低的相对量，因此，也可用绝对危险度降低率除以对照组事件发生率来计算，RRR=100 * (CER−EER)/CER。
- 比值比（OR）：试验组事件发生比与对照组事件发生比的比值。OR>1 或 RR>1，表示与暴露有关的不良结局风险增加；RR=1 或 OR=1，表示有暴露史的人发生不良结局的风险和没有暴露史的人无差别；RR＜1 或 OR＜1，表示暴露于可疑因素的人发生不良结局风险小于无暴露的人，提示该暴露具有保护作用。RR/OR 离 1 越远则关联性越强。

- 需治人数（NNT）：与对照组相比，防止额外一例危险结局发生所需要治疗的人数。NNT 是绝对危险度降低的倒数：NNT＝1/ARR。NNT 的 95%可信区间（CI）可利用 ARR 的 95%可信区间来计算，即 NNT 95% CI 下限值＝1/ARR 上限值，NNT95% CI 上限值＝1/ARR 下限值。NNT 越大，则治疗效果越小。

- 需危害人数（NNH）：是指对患者采取某种防治措施，比对照组多发生 1 例不良反应需要治疗的患者数。NNH＝1/|EER－CER|＝1/ARI。NNT 与 NNH 的意思一样，NNT 一般指一种治疗性干预而 NNH 指不利作用或危害因素。

- 获益与危害似然比（LHH）：反映了治疗措施给受试者带来的收益与危害的比例：LHH＝（1/NNT÷1/NNH）。LHH＞1，利大于弊；反之 LHH＜1 时，弊大于利。

B. 分析计量资料的常用统计学指标：

- 均数（Mean）：对服从正态分布的计量资料，均数是最常用的反映数据集中趋势的统计学指标，Mean＝一组数据之和/该组数据的个数。

- 均数差（MD）：在治疗性研究中某结局指标干预前后均数的差值。

- 加权均数差（WMD）：通常用于基于 RCT 的 Meta 分析，合并来自不同研究的效应量时，按照不同研究样本量的大小给予其对应的研究结果一个权重系数，样本量越大权重系数越大，该研究对合并后结果的影响也越大，这一过程称为加权，最终合并后的均数差则称为加权均数差。

- 标准化均数差（SMD）：通常也用于基于 RCT 的 Meta 分析。有时不同研究测量同一结局指标时采用了不同的测量方法（如采用了不同的量表），此时就不能简单地将不同研究的得分合并，而需要先将不同研究的得分"标准化"处理，方法是用均数差除以对应的标准差，再进行合并。

（2）疗效的精确度：无论研究的样本量有多大，也只是从总体抽取的样本，这就需要通过统计学的方法以样本统计量推断总体参数。疗效的精确度反映样本推断总体的可信程度，常用可信区间表示。可信区间是按预先给定的概率（通常为 95%或 99%）去估计总体参数的可能范围。例如，95%CI 就是该区间有 95%的概率包含了被估计的总体参数。样本量越大，抽样误差越小，CI 就越窄，精确度越高。

6. 重要性评价任务

互动 6.4：TPS

教师：请各位同学根据 Beausoleil M 的文献,用 10 分钟的时间完成工作表 2,并与同桌讨论。

工作表 2：治疗性研究的重要性评价

研究结果是什么?		
研究结局		
结　　局	Lactobacilli 组 $N=44$	安慰剂组 $N=45$
AAD 发生		
AAD 未发生		
OR		95%CI
RR		95%CI
NNT		95%CI

学生：(完成工作表 2 并讨论)

教师：时间到,有谁愿意把自己的答案写在黑板上并说明 OR 值和 NNT 的计算方法? 同时,为我们解释一下 OR 和 NNT 的含义。

学生：(回答问题)

教师：你们是否算对了呢? 请按下表核对自己的答案。

工作表 2：治疗性研究的重要性评价(核对)

研究结果是什么?(研究证据的重要性评价)		
研究结局		
结　　局	Lactobacilli 组 $N=44$	安慰剂组 $N=45$
AAD 发生	7	16
AAD 未发生	37	29
OR	0.34	95%CI(0.125,0.944)
RR	0.45	95%CI
NNT	5	95%CI

7. 相关性评价

能把研究的结果应用于我当前的患者吗？在此之前,你必须考虑下列问题

（1）自己患者的情况是否与研究中的患者相似？

（2）我的患者是否符合研究纳入标准？如果没有,是否有令人信服的理由说明这些结果不适用于我的患者？

（3）是否考虑到所有重要的临床结局？

（4）治疗措施对患者潜在的利弊和花费如何？

（5）回到你的患者,把证据和自己的医学素养结合起来运用。充分关注你的患者,结合他们的需求,给出你的治疗建议,考虑治疗相关费用和副作用,帮助他们决定是否服用益生菌。请完成工作表 3。

工作表 3：治疗性研究的相关性评价

研究证据适用于当前的患者吗？（相关性评价原则）
当前患者的情况与研究中的患者是否相似？
治疗性证据的可行性如何？
是否已考虑到所有临床重要结局（包括阳性的和阴性的结局）？
治疗措施对患者潜在的利弊和花费如何？

李红梅

Chapter 6

Critical Appraisal of Therapeutic Studies

Part I　Teaching Requirements

This session is about how to appraise therapeutic study critically, which aims to help students learn about the validity, importance and relevance of the articles on health care interventions and help students make independent interpretations and judgements about the findings from these trial reports. Students will know about that critical evaluations of research report findings are fundamental to the practice of EBM.

1. Teaching aims

The aim is to show how to improve the ability of identification of effective health interventions by using evidence-based techniques to frame answerable therapeutic questions, search for the literature and critically appraise therapeutic studies.

2. Learning objectives

After completing this session, students should be able to:

(1) Frame answerable therapeutic questions.

(2) Describe the 3 main appraisal aspects (validity/importance/relevance) of therapeutic studies.

(3) List different types of bias that threaten the validity of an RCT.

(4) Understand the importance of clinical significance, confidence interval and the different measures of treatment effect and effect size (OR/RR).

(5) Calculate the RR, NNT from trial results reporting outcomes.

（6）Know the considerations when applying the results of particular studies to individual patients.

3. Teaching methods

This session will use lecture, PPT presentation and interactive teaching method. Interactive teaching techniques include TPR, instructor storytelling and TPS.

4. Reading materials

（1）Beausoleil M. Effect of a fermented milk combining *Lactobacillus acidophilus* Cl1285 and *Lactobacillus casei* in the prevention of antibiotic-associated diarrhea: a randomized, double-blind, placebo-controlled trial. Can J Gastroenterol, 2007,21(11): 732 – 736.

（2）Guyatt G H, Sackett D L, Cook D J, et al. Users' guides to the medical literature: II. How to use an article about therapy or prevention: A. Are the results of the study valid?. Jama, 1993, 270(21): 2598 – 2601.

Part II　Teaching Design — 2 periods（80 minutes）

Teaching design of "Critical Appraisal of Therapeutic Studies"

No.	Content	Interactive technique/ teaching techniques	Descriptions	Time (minutes)
1	Review	Interaction 6.1: TPR	Using TPR to go over the lessons last week.	10
2	Introduction to validity	PPT presentation	Introduce the following contents: the reference scope of "therapy" and "therapeutic question"; the best evidence for therapeutic questions; influencing factors to therapeutic results and the solutions.	15
3	A clinical story	Interaction 6.2: Instructor storytelling	Instructor illustrates the story of a real case, asking students to think about how to deal with it using EBM principles.	10

（**continued**）

No.	Content	Interactive technique/teaching techniques	Descriptions	Time（minutes）
4	Validity appraisal task	Interaction 6.3：TPS	Introduce the critical appraisal worksheet of validity（see Appendix Ⅳ）. Ask student to read the paper by Beausoleil M，and fill out the worksheet，then discuss in pairs，then，share in the class.	15
5	Importance appraisal	PPT presentation	Introduce importance appraisal aspect of therapeutic study. Focus on measures of treatment effect，precision and confidence interval.	15
6	Importance appraisal task	Interaction 6.4：TPS	Students complete calculation task based on Beausoleil M study.	10
7	Relevance appraisal	PPT presentation	Introduce some questions for students to consider before applying the results of a study to your patient. Remind students of finishing their worksheet 3 and KWL chart.	5

Part III   Teaching Contents

1. Review：using TPR to go over the lessons last week

Interaction 6.1：TPR

Teacher：Good morning, everyone! Let's begin the class with your KWL chart. Please take a quick glance at your KWL chart. Two minutes later，I will ask some True/False questions about what you've learnt and you need to give me a response. If you think the answer is true, please stand up; if you think the answer is false，keep sitting down.

Now, are you ready?

(1) The three essential components of EBM include evidence, doctor and medical facilities. True or False?

Students: (response)

Teacher: (2) One of the important basic elements of evidence classification and grading is research designs in clinical epidemiology. True or False?

Students: (response)

Teacher: (3) The first scholar to define the concept of 'evidence-based medicine' is Archie Cochrane. True or False?

Students: (response)

Teacher: (4) Formulating an evidence-based clinical practice question, you don't need to consider the outcomes. True or False?

Students: (response)

Teacher: (5) Formulating an evidence-based clinical practice question, you need to consider PICO. True or False?

Students: (response)

Teacher: (6) EBM is clinical practice based on best evidence, clinical expertise and patients' values. True or False?

Students: (response)

Teacher: (7) 6S approach classifies evidence resources into 6 categories, eg. system, summaries, synopses, syntheses, synopses of studies, studies. True or False?

Students: (response)

Teacher: (8) According to EBM practice 5As, searching evidence is the second step. True or False?

Students: (response)

Teacher: (9) The goal of evidence classification and grading is to utilize evidence effectively. True or False?

Students: (response)

Teacher: (10) Evidence classification and grading is based on research design. True or False?

Students：（response）

Teacher：（11）The Evidence Pyramid is a 8-level system, which includes animal research and *in vitro* study for the first time. True or False?

Students：（response）

Teacher：（12）Evidence could be classified into two categories: primary research evidence and secondary research evidence. True or False?

Students：（response）

2. Introduction

Clinical Practice, in a sense, is a process of answering a series of questions and making decisions. The practice of EBM emphasizes using the best available research evidence in clinical decision making. The best evidence usually comes from well designed and implemented poems （being patient-oriented that matters） researches. The results from good researches can reflect the real situation of the subjects （i.e. internal validity） and can be generalized to the whole as well （i.e. external validity）.Today we are going to learn how to identify a good therapeutic research.

（1）The reference scope of "therapy" and "therapeutic question": Therapy is the attempted remediation of a health problem, usually following a diagnosis. In the medical field, it is usually synonymous with treatment. The words care, therapy, treatment, and intervention overlap in a semantic field, and thus they can be synonymous depending on context.

Therapy mostly refers to individual intervention, such as drug therapy, surgery, rehabilitation, nursing, psychotherapy, life style change （i.e. smoking cessation, exercise therapy, diet therapy）, sometime it also refers to social activity （i.e. health education plan, bibliotherapy, mass intervention, prevention and control, disease screening）.

Therapeutic question refers to the effectiveness and safety of a intervention, accounting for a large proportion in all the clinical questions. Clinical task is to select cost-effective treatments that do more good than harm for patients. Therapeutic study is designed to answer therapeutic question.

(2) The best evidence for therapeutic questions: What is the best evidence to answer therapeutic question? Please go over the Evidence Pyramid (see in Chapter 3). In this hierarchy structure, different types of clinical research or sources of information provide varying levels of evidence according to their research designs. As a result, for healthcare interventions, generally speaking, systematic reviews (SR) and Meta-analysis, large RCTs are considered to be the "gold standard". However, regardless of the type and source of reviews or studies, all evidence requires critical appraisal. For example, a high quality SR, with definitive results, and based on the homogeneity individual trials, represents the highest level of evidence. Large RCTs with definitive results (a result with confidence intervals that do not overlap the threshold clinically significant effect) are better than RCTs with non-definitive results (point estimate suggests a clinically significant effect but with confidence intervals overlapping the threshold for this effect). A well-designed large cohort study might provide more valid evidence than a randomized-controlled study with serious methodological flaws.

(3) Influencing factors to therapeutic researches and the solutions

A. Chance and bias: Chance refers to the difference between the measured value (observed value) and the true value caused by probability, which can lead to random error. Its effects can be estimated by statistical methods, but there is no directionality, that is, the measured value is randomly higher or lower than the truth value. Random error is inevitable in sampling research. We can only control it in a certain range. Bias, or systematic error, refers to the deviation between the observed value and the true value caused by researchers, equipments or research methods. Unlike chance, bias always makes research results above or below the true value, so it is directional. It is difficult to estimate the effects of bias quantitatively in a study, but the direction of bias is easier to be predicted. Different types of bias may occur during the study, such as selection bias, measurement bias/detection bias/ascertainment bias. Researchers could avoid selection bias to the greatest extent mainly by strict design, and random allocation.

B. Sample size: Sample size directly reflects the degree of the influence caused by chance. It is more possibly affected by chance for small sample studies, so they tend to give false positive results or false negative results. The larger the sample size, the less affection by chance, the more closer to the truth of results.

C. Compliance: Compliance refers to the objective response degree of the subjects in accordance with the research requirements. In clinical trials of new drugs, compliance can be defined as the extent to which the subject takes the test drug in accordance with the prescribed dosage and course of treatment. The compliance of subjects is closely related to the quality of test results. Noncompliance or poor compliance is the most common cause of treatment failure, and noncompliance is very common in clinical trials of new drugs. According to statistics, subjects with complete compliance, poor compliance and complete noncompliance accounted for about 1/3 each. Measures to improve compliance include: strengthening patient compliance education, choosing simple and feasible treatment plan when it is possible, improving medical staff's service attitude and medical technology level, and dealing with adverse drug reactions in time.

D. Regression to the mean: Regression to the mean refers to the trend that for some of the patients with abnormal indicators, even if they don't get treated, in the subsequent continuous measurement, these indicators are close to the normal. This phenomenon may be caused by the fluctuation of the measurement value around the mean value, or the physiological fluctuation of the measurement index, rather than by the intervention. Regression to the mean can give the illusion that treatment is effective. In the same condition, at different time, getting mean value of multiple measurements to the indicator of the same individual can reduce the influence on the results.

E. Contamination and co-intervention: Contamination refers to the fact that the subjects of control group accept the treatment of experimental group consciously or unconsciously. Contamination reduces possible differences between the experimental group and the control group. Co-Intervention means that subjects in the experimental group or control group receive additional treatment similar to the experimental intervention, thereby artificially affecting the efficacy of the experimental intervention. Contamination and Co-intervention can be avoided by double-blind or triple-blind design.

F. Hawthorne effect: Hawthorne effect refers to some effects caused by researchers and subjects. In a study, researchers may pay more attention to those subjects they are interested in, and the subjects may improve their behavior consciously or unconsciously when they have been paid more attention to, thus may exaggerate the efficacy of intervention. The way to avoid the Hawthorne effect is to set up a control group with a double-blind or triple-blind design.

3. A clinical story

Interaction 6.2 : Instructor storytelling

The instructor illustrates a story of a real case, asking the students to think about how to deal with it using EBM principles.

Teacher: I would like to tell you a real story of mine. My friend's mother is a 70-year-old highly-functional lady, but recently she was sent to the emergency room after a fall in her home. Medical workup identified a right femur fracture. The doctor recommended urgent repair and preoperative antibiotics. My friend asked me for suggestion. Because I have read some articles about the possibility of diarrhea as a side effect of the antibiotics especially for the elderly people, so I told her to ask the doctor whether using fermented milk with lactobacillus or some other probiotic products would prevent this side effect. The doctor didn't give us a definite answer, so if I wanted to find out the answer, if I wanted to practice EBM by myself, how would I do? Could you please tell me the steps of practicing EBM?

Student 1: Ask an answerable question. Acquire the evidence. Appraise the evidence. Apply the evidence. Assess the after-effect.

Teacher: Great! Let's do the first step: ask an answerable question. Here, I have three questions, which one is the best?

A: What is the best treatment for diarrhea?

B: For patients taking antibiotics, will using probiotics at the same time be helpful in preventing diarrhea?

C: Can probiotics prevent the elderly hospitalized patients from antibiotics-associated diarrhea?

Students 2：C.

Teacher：Good! the second step also provides three options about search strategy. If we choose PubMed, which is the best to address the clinical question?

A：diarrhea AND best treatment Limited to free full text.

B：diarrhea AND probiotics AND elderly AND female AND adult Limited to English.

C：antibiotics AND diarrhea AND probiotics Limited to meta-analysis, systematic review, randomized controlled trial.

Students 3：C.

Teacher：Good job! We use C to search PubMed. We may get many study evidence, including meta-analysis, systematic review, randomized controlled trial. Now we come to the third step of EBM practicing — appraisal. How shall we appraise a therapeutic evidence? Here I have a critical appraisal worksheet for you.

4. Validity appraisal task

Introduce the critical appraisal worksheet of validity. Ask student to read the paper by Beausoleil M, and fill in the worksheet, then discuss the result in pairs, and share it in the class.

Interaction 6.3：TPS

Teacher：After searching the clinical question, we got retrieval results. In our retrieval results, there are the highest level of evidence (SR, META) and also there are many primary researches. Before applying them to supporting clinical decision, they are needed to be appraised. As for SR, Meta-analysis, we will talk about them later. Today, we will focus on primary research appraisal. Beausoleil M's paper is one of those primary research. Are the results of this study valid? Please read the paper and fill in Worksheet 1 which is usually used to assess the validity of studies. Then discuss the result in pairs, and share it in the class. You have 15 minutes.

Worksheet 1: Validity appraisal of therapeutic studies

Are the results of the study valid?	Yes	No	Not clear
1. Were the subjects (patients) randomly assigned to experimental group and control group?			
2. Was the group allocation concealed?			
3. Were the groups comparable at baseline?			
4. Were patients, health workers, and study personnel "blind" to treatment?			
5. Was follow-up sufficiently long and complete?			
6. Were all patients properly accounted for and attributed at its conclusion?			
7. Aside from the experimental intervention, were the groups treated equally?			

Students: (read and discuss)

Teacher: Time is up. Let's check your answers.

Number 1, were the patients randomly assigned? Yes! The paper reported that patients were randomly assigned. But it didn't elaborate on how the randomization is conducted, so it's hard to tell if the study was really randomizaion. Can you tell me what randomization is? Why randomization is so important?

Student: Randomization is a random sampling procedure to reduce bias.

Teacher: Yes. Randomization is an important method and basic principle of clinical research, including that subjects are randomly sampled and randomly assigned to intervention group and control group. Selection bias is due to certain difference in characteristics of groups, making groups lack of comparability. Using appropriate methods, such as computer-generated random numbers, randomly assigning subjects to the control and experimental groups will eliminate potential bias. Using alternate grouping or out-patient number/hospital number grouping, investigators may also subvert the randomization. In addition, inadequate allocation concealment is also an important source of bias, so investigators should be kept unknown to the allocation program.

Now, let's look at number 2. Was group allocation concealed? Yes or no? We don't know. The article did not provide enough information to help us determine whether or not its allocation was concealed. Why is allocation concealed important?

Students: Prevent investigators from subverting the randomization process.

Teacher: Correct, we discussed it in Number 1.

Number 3, were the groups similar at the start of the trial? Were all baseline characteristics similar across groups? Yes, the baseline characteristics were shown in table 1. It's worth noticing that the placebo group took more laxatives and beta-lactams. You may think about whether this difference will affect the results of the experiment or not. Why do we need to look at baseline?

Student: To maintain balance and comparability between groups.

Teacher: Good! let's look at number 4. Were patients, health workers, and study personnel "blind" to treatment? The patients were blinded. Both groups were given drugs that looked the same, tasted the same and had the same texture. However, although this was a double-blind trial, it was not clear who the other blind subjects were. Why is blind so important?

Student: To reduce subjective influences from the researchers or the subjects.

Teacher: Yes, for example, Hawthorne effect. What else? Double blinding can also reduce performance bias and detection bias. Performance bias is due to the different understanding to the allocated interventions by participants and personnel during the study. In this situation neither the patients nor the investigators were aware of which treatment the participant was given. Double blinding also prevents people from being against placebo effects. For researches with subjective outcomes such as pain, double-blind is particularly important. Where outcome assessment differs systematically between comparison groups, detection bias may occur. Outcome assessment should be blinded, where possible.

Number 5, follow-up, was follow-up complete and sufficiently long? Where can we find the evidence in this paper?

Student: Follow-up was complete. They had data for all patients in the study which lasted up to 21 days after the last administration of antibiotics.

Teacher: Ideally, all subjects should complete the experiment and obtain experiment data. If patients drop out of trials because of side effects, and their data are not analyzed, the efficacy of testing intervention may be overestimated. Generally speaking, the withdraw rate should be controlled within 10%, and under special circumstances, the withdrawal rate should not exceed 20%. In addition, we should ensure sufficient follow-up time to observe clinical effects.

Number 6, were patients properly grouped for analysis and calculation? Was the principle of intention-to-treat analysis followed? Yes, this study reported that both primary and secondary outcomes were analyzed based on intention-to-treat principle. But what is intention-to-treat analysis?

Intention-to-treat (ITT) analysis refers to all subjects (including drug suspension or taking other treatment) should be taken into final statistical analysis, and be statistically analized in their initially assigned group. Observational studies have shown that treatment outcomes are generally worse for those who drop out than those who complete the trial, so not including these subjects in the analysis can lead to an overestimate of treatment outcomes. Intention-to-treat analysis is mainly used to prevent the attrition bias which is systematically different between comparison groups because of participants withdrawing from the study, or because of protocol violations.

Number 7, aside from the experimental intervention, were the groups treated equally?

Student: Yes.

Teacher: Why we need equal treatment?

Student: Keep balance between groups.

Teacher: Great! to avoid confounding bias. Confounding is the existence of one or more external factors that confuse or interfere with the relationship between exposure and outcome. So far, we have finished the validity appraisal of therapeutic studies. Please amend your validity worksheet according to the following table and remember the 7 aspects of validity. Next，we will come to the importance appraisal.

Worksheet 1：Validity appraisal of therapeutic studies（check）

Are the results of the study valid?	Yes	No	Not clear
1. Were the subjects（patients）randomly assigned to experimental group and control group?	√		
2. Was group allocation concealed?			√
3. Were the groups similar at the start of the trial?	√		
4. Were patients，health workers，and study personnel "blind" to treatment?	√		
5. Was follow-up sufficiently long and complete?	√		
6. Were all patients properly accounted for and attributed at its conclusion?	√		
7. Aside from the experimental intervention，were the groups treated equally?	√		

5. Importance appraisal（What is the result? How precise is it? Can it change my clinical decision?）

The importance appraisal should be on the basis of validity. The importance appraisal includes evaluating the effect size and the precision.

（1）Measures of treatment effect：In EBM，two categories of statistical effect size are commonly used to evaluate the treatment effect of a intervention. One is applied to analyze categorical variables（e.g., disease incidence and mortality，etc.），and the other is applied to analyze numerical variables（e.g., blood pressure，blood sugar level，height，weight，etc.）.

A. The commonly-used statistical effect size for categorical variables：Suppose a parallel randomized placebo-controlled trial，with a long enough follow-up period，is designed to prevent one adverse event（e.g., death），and the effect of treatment is reflected in two outcomes（event occurrence/event non-occurrence），then the following indicators can be calculated.

- Control group event rate（CER）：CER＝The incidence of an event in the control group.
- Experimental group event rate（EER）：EER＝The incidence of an

event in the experimental group.

- Absolute risk reduction (ARR): The difference between the control group and the experimental group in the incidence of adverse outcome event, ARR=CER−EER.
- Relative risk (RR): The ratio of event rate in the experimental group to that in the control group, RR=EER/CER. RR=1 is the null value or no difference.
- Relative risk reduction (RRR): It is related to the relative risk and can be calculated by the following formula, RRR=1−RR. The relative risk reduction rate reflects the relative amount of event reduction in the experimental group and the control group. Therefore, it can also be calculated by RRR=100 * (CER−EER)/CER.
- Odds Ratio (OR): It is the ratio of the odds of an event occurring in experimental group to the odds of it occurring in control group. OR>1 or RR>1 indicates an increased risk of adverse outcomes associated with exposure; RR=1 or OR=1, indicates the same risk of adverse outcomes between people with exposure and people without exposure; RR<1 or OR<1 indicates that the risk of adverse outcomes in people exposed to suspicious factors is lower than that in people without exposure. This suggests that the exposure has a protective effect. The farther RR/OR is from 1, the stronger the correlation is.
- Number needed to treat (NNT): It is the number of patients you need to treat to prevent one additional bad outcome. NNT is the inverse of the absolute risk reduction, NNT = 1/ARR. The 95% (confidence interval, CI) for the NNT can be calculated by simply inverting and exchanging the limits of a 95% CI for the ARR. That is NNT 95% CI lower limit = 1/upper limit of ARR, NNT 95% CI upper limit = 1/lower limit of ARR. The higher the NNT is, the less effective the treatment is.
- Number needed to harm (NNH): It is the number needed to cause harm to one more patient from the therapy. NNH=1/|EER−CER|=1/ARI.

NNT is similar to NNH, where NNT usually refers to a therapeutic intervention and NNH refers to a detrimental effect or risk factor.

- Benefit-to-harm likelihood ratio (LHH): This index reflects the ratio of benefit to harm given to subjects by treatment, LHH=(1/NNT÷ 1/NNH). LHH > 1, the advantages outweigh the disadvantages; conversely, LHH<1 does more harm than good.

B. The commonly-used statistical effect size for numerical variable:

- Mean: for numerical data of obeying normal distribution. Mean is most commonly used to reflect the central tendency of data. Mean=the sum of a group of data divided by the number of that group of data.

- Mean Difference (MD): In therapeutic studies, MD refers to the Mean Difference before and after intervention of a certain outcome indicator.

- Weighted Mean Difference (WMD): It is usually used for Meta-analysis based on RCT. When we combine the effect sizes from different studies, the corresponding research results are given a weight coefficient according to the sample size of different studies. The larger the sample size, the greater the weight coefficient, the greater the influence of the research on the combined results. This process is called weighting, and the final pooled mean difference is called weighted mean difference.

- Standardized mean difference (SMD): It is also commonly used in Meta-analysis. based on RCT. Sometimes different studies adopt different measurement methods when we measure the same outcome index (for example, different scales are adopted). At this time, the scores of different studies cannot be simply pooled. Instead, the scores of different studies need to be "standardized" first. The method is taking the mean difference divided by the corresponding standard deviation first, and then synthesizing.

(2) Precision of efficacy: No matter how large the sample size of a study is, it's just a sample from the whole. We need to infer the true value of the whole by using statistical methods. The precision of efficacy reflects the reliability of the inference from the samples to the whole, which is often expressed as a CI. CI is an estimate of the possible range of true value of the whole with a given probability (usually 95% or 99%)。For example, a 95% CI is a 95% probability that the interval contains the estimated true value of

the whole. The larger the sample size, the smaller the sampling error, the narrower the CI, and the higher the precision.

6. Importance appraisal task

Interaction 6.4 : TPS

Teacher: Please fill in worksheet 2, based on Beausoleil M study. Then discuss it with your deskmates. We have 10 minutes.

Worksheet 2: Importance appraisal of therapeutic studies

What are the results?		
Outcomes according to study group		
Outcome	Lactobacilli group $N=44$	Placebo group $N=45$
AAD occurrence		
AAD absent		
OR		95%CI
RR		95%CI
NNT		95%CI

Students: (completing and discussing)

Teacher: Time is up. I would like to ask some volunteers to write their answers on the blackboard, and tell us how you calculated OR and NNT. Also, tell us what OR and NNT mean.

Student: (answer questions)

Teacher: Did you get right results? Please check whether your answers are the same as the following worksheet indicates.

Worksheet 2: Importance appraisal of therapeutic studies (check)

What are the results?		
Outcomes according to study group		
Outcome	Lactobacilli group $N=44$	Placebo group $N=45$
AAD occurrence	7	16
AAD absent	37	29
OR	0.34	95%CI (0.125, 0.944)
RR	0.45	95%CI
NNT	5	95%CI

7. Relevance appraisal

Can I apply the results to my patient? The following questions need to be considered before applying the results of a study to your patient:

(1) Are the patients in the study similar to my population of interest?

(2) Does my patient match the study inclusion criteria? If not, are there compelling reasons why the results should not be applied to my patient?

(3) Are all the clinically important outcomes considered?

(4) Are the likely treatment benefits worth the potential harm and costs?

(5) Return to the patient and integrate that evidence with clinical expertise, patient preferences and apply it to practice. Think about your patient, her goals, your treatment recommendations for her, the cost and adverse effects, and help her decide whether to start taking the probiotics. Please finish Worksheet 3.

Worksheet 3: Relevance appraisal of therapeutic studies

Can these results by applied to my patient care?
Is your patient similar to those in the study?
Is the treatment feasible in your setting?
Are all clinical important outcomes considered? (both positive and negative outcomes)
Are the likely treatment benefits worth the potential harms and costs?

Li Hongmei

第 7 章

危险因素与病因学研究的严格评价

第一部分　教　学　要　求

此教学环节首先介绍病因学的相关概念。其次介绍病因学研究设计类型和证据的评价方法。着重让学生通过阅读经典文献以及练习，掌握病因证据的严格评价。

1. 教学目的

讨论病因学的相关概念、研究设计类型和危险因素与病因学研究的严格评价方法。

2. 学习目标

通过此环节的学习，学生能够：

（1）理解病因学的相关概念。

（2）知晓病因研究设计的类型及其论证强度。

（3）对病因学研究进行严格评价。

3. 教学方法

此环节采用讲授法、PPT 演示和互动教学法，互动教学技术包括思考时段、波浪和评价任务等。

4. 阅读材料

（1）Straus S E，Richardson W S，Glasziu P，et al. Evidence-based medicine：how to practice and teach EBM. 3th ed. Singapore：Elsevier（Singapore）Pte Ltd.，2006.

（2）Lily A. Arya，Deborah L. Myers，et al. Dietary caffeine intake and the risk for detrusor instability：a case-control study. Obstetrics &

Gynecology，2000，96(1)：85 - 89.

第二部分　教学设计——2 课时(80 分钟)

"危险因素与病因学研究的严格评价"教学设计表

序号	内　容	互动技术/教学技术	描　　　　述	时间(分钟)
1	课程概要	PPT 演示	复习治疗性研究评价的三个方面,通过 PPT 简要介绍本章课程的内容和安排	5
2	病因概述	PPT 演示 互动 7.1：思考时段	提出问题,让学生们思考,引出病因和危险因素概念,介绍病因学研究及其目的	5
3	病因学研究类型及论证强度	PPT 演示	介绍病因学研究类型并分析病因论证强度	10
4	介绍临床案例	PPT 演示 互动 7.2：TPS	提出临床案例与阅读材料,让学生思考循证医学实践的步骤	10
5	病因学研究的真实性评价	互动 7.3：波浪 PPT 演示	使用波浪活动将学生分组(5 人/组),学生阅读 Lily A 的文献,讨论并完成病因研究评价工作表1	25
6	病因学研究的重要性评价及相关性评价	互动 7.4：评价任务	学生完成证据的重要性和相关性评价任务	25

第三部分　教　学　内　容

1. 本章概要

课程主要包括 3 个方面的内容：

(1)病因概述。

(2)病因学研究设计的类型(病例对照研究、队列研究和随机对照试验)及其论证强度。

(3)病因学研究的严格评价。

2. 病因学概述

提出问题,让学生们思考,引出病因相关概念。

互动 7.1：思考时段

教师： 作为医务人员，每天都可能面临各种各样关于疾病的问题，患者除了关注疾病的治疗外，常常也会问及"我为什么会得这个病""有什么因素导致我得这个病"。正确回答这些问题不仅和医师的临床决策相关，也有助于医师和患者及其家属的有效沟通和交流。此外，危险因素的问题常常也是公众所关心的问题。例如，住在水力发电线路附近会增加患癌症的风险吗？如果你被问到这些问题，你的答案是什么？

学生： 不会。

教师： 另一个问题，长期服用他汀类药物会致癌吗？

学生： 也许会。

教师： 真的吗？有证据吗？

学生： 没有。

教师： 接触铝会导致阿尔茨海默病吗？

学生： 会。

教师： 你真是这么认为的吗？为什么？

学生： 我不知道。也许是……

教师： 同型半胱氨酸升高会导致冠状动脉疾病吗？

学生： 我不知道。

教师： 上面提到的问题，有些是关于疾病危险因素的，有些是关于病因的，要回答这些问题，需要进行病因学研究，或者对已经进行的研究进行严格评价。我们先来澄清几个概念：什么是病因或致病因素？什么是危险因素？什么是病因学研究及其目的？请大家思考，并与同桌讨论一下。

（1）病因或致病因素：指作用于人体后在一定的条件下可导致疾病发生的外界客观存在的生物、物理、化学和社会等有害因素，或人体本身的不良心理状态及遗传缺陷等因素。

（2）危险因素：指与疾病发生及其消长有一定因果关系的因素，但尚无充分依据能阐明其明确的致病效应。但这些因素存在时，其相关疾病（事件）发生率会相应增高；而当其被消除后，该疾病（事件）发生率随之下降。例如，吸烟、高血压、高胆固醇血症等为缺血性心脏病的危险因素。

（3）病因学研究：关于致病因素或危险因素与疾病之间的因果关系的研究。研究干预措施引起的不良反应，实质上也是确定因果关系，也属于病因学研究。

（4）病因学研究及其目的：

A. 弄清病因、估计危害程度。

B. 针对病因和危险因素进行干预（包括预防和治疗），以控制疾病。

3. 病因学研究设计及论证强度

理想状态下，要回答关于病因的问题，基于多个随机对照试验或高质量的队列研究的系统评价或 Meta 分析结果能提供最好的病因证据，但这方面的证据还不是太多，需要我们对单个的临床试验进行评价。

病因学研究方法按其因果论证强度高低排序为：多个随机对照试验的系统评价、单个随机对照试验、队列研究、病例对照研究、描述性研究，详见下表。

病因学研究的论证强度

设　计	开始点	结果评价	优　势	缺　点	论证强度
随机对照试验	暴露状态	不良事件	具前瞻性 可比性好	伦理问题 可行性差	＋＋＋＋
队列研究	暴露状态	不良事件	多具前瞻性 设有对照	非随机	＋＋＋
病例对照研究	不良事件	暴露状态	样本量需要较少 不存在伦理问题	回忆偏倚	＋＋
描述性研究	暴露状态	不良事件		无对照	＋

（1）随机对照试验：随机对照试验中，受试对象被随机分配到试验组和对照组。随机分配使可能影响结局的因素（包括已知的和未知的因素）在组间均衡分布，从而消除未知混杂因素的影响，且研究者能主动控制暴露因素或治疗措施。这是其论证强度高的原因之一。

但有两方面原因限制了采用随机对照试验研究不良反应或暴露因素的致病效应。一方面，当我们认为某种干预或暴露因素可能有害时，将受试者随机分配入试验组和对照组并接受可能有害的暴露，存在伦理问题。另一方面，干预措施的不良反应少见、严重和潜伏期长时，研究需要极大的样本量和长时期的观察，其可行性较差。

（2）队列研究：队列研究按是否接触某暴露因素将受试人群自然分为两个群体，随访一定的时期后，比较各群体某疾病发生情况的差异。队列研究与随机对照试验的区别在于，受试对象的暴露与否不是随机分配形成的，而是由受试人群自行决定或自然形成。由于暴露因素自然存在于人群中，研究者无法主动控制,因此队列研究易受到混杂因素的影响。

（3）病例对照研究：是一种回顾性研究方法,是对出现某种不良反应的病例和没有出现某种不良反应的病例,回顾性地调查过去或最近有无接受某种治疗措施或接触暴露,再比较两组暴露的情况。这适用于少见和潜伏期长的疾病的研究,耗时短,省钱省力,对患者无害,没有伦理问题,可同时探索多种暴露和研究结局之间的可能关系。然而由于信息完全基于回忆的基础,这种方法容易产生回忆性偏倚,另外,也更易受到混杂因素的影响。因此,病例对照研究常常只能推导可能的病因,而不能验证病因。

4. 临床案例

提出临床案例,启发学生思考如何应用循证医学的原理解决问题。

> **互动 7.2：TPS**
>
> **教师**：假设你是一个临床医生,这天,诊所来了这样一个患者：45 岁的妇女,她抱怨在过去两年多,发生急迫性尿失禁情况越来越严重,严重影响了她的生活质量。她有三次怀孕史（她的急迫性尿失禁与这个有关）,其中两次分娩时用了产钳。她偶尔在晚上入睡困难时服用氯拉西泮,没有服用其他药物史和吸烟史,每天摄入咖啡 750 毫升（约 708 克）。当她在截石位咳嗽时可见尿漏,其余临床检查无异常。排尿后残余尿量为 20 毫升,尿液分析无异常。她最近在报纸上读到,咖啡因会导致尿失禁,她想知道这是否是真的,或者是否有其他因素导致她的问题。
>
> 谁能回答这个患者的问题？如果不能回答,应该怎么做呢？你们能告诉我实践循证医学的步骤吗？
>
> **学生 1**：提出问题,查找证据,评价证据,应用证据,后效评价。
>
> **教师**：非常好！让我们从第一步开始,提出临床问题。还记得临床问题的结果吗？
>
> **学生 2**：PICO。
>
> **教师**：患者想知道喝咖啡是否会导致尿失禁,或使尿失禁加重,这是一个关于病因的问题,所以,问题的结构应该变成 PECO,E 是暴露因素。现在,我请 2 位同学把各自的临床问题写在黑板上。
>
> **学生 3**：对于 45 岁的女性,喝咖啡会导致尿失禁吗？
>
> **学生 4**：对于尿失禁的女性,每天摄入 750 毫升咖啡会增加患尿失禁的风险吗？

教师：好，现在我们有了两个问题，大家觉得哪一个更好一点？第二个，对，P是尿失禁的女性，E是每天摄入较多的咖啡，C为不摄入或少量摄入，O是尿失禁或者尿失禁加重。现在我们进行第二步，检索证据。采用策略"urge incontinence AND（coffee OR caffeine）"来检索，可以检索到不同级别的证据。请问各位，对于病因学问题来说，证据级别最高的是什么？

学生：系统评价或Meta分析

教师：好的，如果我们检索到了下面四篇文献，请你们按照证据的级别进行排序。请思考并和同桌讨论，5分钟后我请同学把他们的答案写在黑板上。

（1）Coffee and caffeine intake and risk of urinary incontinence：a Meta-analysis of observational studies.

（2）Prevalence and risk factors for urinary incontinence in Italy：a cross-sectional study.

（3）Prevalence and risk factors for urine leakage in a racially and ethnically diverse population of adults：a cohort study.

（4）Is caffeine intake associated with urinary incontinence in Japanese adults：a case-control study.

病因学研究证据是按照病因学研究设计的因果论证强度来排序的。也就是说，一项合并所有相关随机试验或队列研究的系统综述/Meta分析可能会为我们提供足够多的患者，以检测甚至罕见的进展事件因而居于最高等级。病因学研究因伦理学限制通常无法设计随机对照试验，因此，大样本的观察性研究如队列研究，是最高级别的原始研究证据，然后是病例对照研究和描述性研究。你们的排序对了吗？

5. 病因学研究的真实性评价

向学生介绍真实性严格评价工作表。请学生阅读Lily A的文献，完成工作表，同桌讨论并与全班分享。

互动7.3：波浪

教师：让我们做一个波浪活动。现在请从1到5报数（每组5人，如果需要每组4人，则从1到4报数，由此类推。假设的班级学生人数为50），请一定要记住自己报的数。

学生：（报数）

教师：很好，现在，所有号码为1的同学请起立，请坐下。所有号码为2的请起立，好，坐下。号码3起立，请坐。号码4请起立，请坐。号码5，请坐。非常好！现在我们请每一组同学依次起立、坐下，像波浪一样，每组同学起立时同时叫出自己的号码，并高举双臂，现在开始。

学生：（做波浪）

教师：我们请相同号码的同学成为一个学习小组，一共是5个组，每组找一张桌子坐下，然后阅读下面的这篇论文并讨论研究的真实性，完成工作表1。

Lily A. Arya, Deborah L. Myers, et al. Dietary caffeine intake and the risk for detrusor instability: a case-control study. Obstetrics & Guynecology, 2000, 96(1): 85 - 89.

学生：（阅读并讨论）

工作表1：病因学研究真实性评价

这个病因学研究真实吗？	是/否/不清楚	引用文献中的表达
(1) 该病因证据是否采用了论证强度高的研究设计方法？		
(2) 试验组和对照组的暴露因素、结局测量方法是否一致？（对结局的测量是客观的吗？是在不知道暴露的情况下测量的吗？）		
(3) 随访时间是否足够长（至结果发生）并完成？		
(4) 病因研究的结果是否符合病因判断条件？ 　—因果时相关系是否明确？ 　—是否存在剂量—效应梯度关系？ 　—暴露因素/干预措施的消长是否与不良反应的消长一致？ 　—不同研究的结果是否一致？ 　—暴露因素/干预措施与不良反应的关系是否符合生物学规律？		

教师：时间到，让我看看你们的作业完成得如何。

(1) 病因证据是否建立在强推理研究设计的基础上？

本文为病例对照研究，推理强度一般。

(2) 两组的治疗/暴露因素结果的测量方法相同吗？

对照组和病例组的参与者都被要求在尿动力学检查前完成48小时的排

尿日记。日记内容包括结构性摄入和排出的情况，并记下液体的种类和量的多少，所摄入的咖啡（记录是否含咖啡因、是速溶的还现磨的）、茶、可乐（记录品牌名称）和可可均用量杯计量。一周后，另一组随机抽样的女性受试者根据日记内容进行完全同样的液体摄入。所有的受试者均不清楚研究假设。再次检查病历以确定潜在的混杂因素，如生育史和吸烟史。

（3）研究患者的随访时间是否足够长（使结果发生）并完成？

研究人群包括 259 名未患尿失禁的女性，她们于 1996 年 10 月至 1998 年 7 月期间，在我们的第三尿动力学中心接受尿失禁的评估。

研究人员要求参与实验的女性记录自己的咖啡摄入量（含咖啡因或不含咖啡因的，速溶或非速溶的）、茶、可乐（包括品牌）、可可。为保证数据的可靠性，在间隔 1 周后通过再测试进行了检验。所有受试者均被纳入其初始分配组进行最终的统计分析。

（4）病因研究的结果是否符合一些病因判断条件？

因为这是一项回顾性病例对照研究，所以因果顺序尚不清楚，需要更多的证据。

6. 如何评价证据的重要性和相关性（适用性）

（1）这种病因学研究结果的重要性如何？

A. 暴露与结局之间的关联有多大？

B. 暴露与结局之间关联评估的精确度如何？

（2）危害性研究的证据真实且重要，它们适用于我们的患者吗？

A. 我们的患者和研究中的患者有什么不同吗？

B. 置于这种暴露因素下，我们的患者可以从中获得利益和危害是什么？

C. 我们的患者对这种治疗的偏好、担忧和期望是什么？

D. 有哪些替代疗法？

互动 7.4：评价任务

教师：（分发病因学评价工作表 2 和工作表 3）请各位同学根据下面这篇文献完成这两个工作表。

Lily A. Arya，Deborah L. Myers，et al. Dietary caffeine intake and the risk for detrusor instability：a case-control study. Obstetrics & Gynecology，2000，96（1）：85-89.

各位同学可以和同桌进行讨论,你们有 25 分钟的时间来完成练习。

学生:(练习和讨论)

工作表 2:病因学研究重要性评价

(1)病因与疾病之间的因果相关强度有多大?

(2)暴露与结局之间关联评估的精确性如何?

结局指标

暴　　露	逼尿肌不稳定组 (N=)	无副尿肌不稳定组 (N=)	OR	95%CI
咖啡因摄取平均值				
高摄入量 (>100 mg/d)				
中等摄入量 (100~400 mg/d)				
低摄入量 (<100 mg/d)				

工作表 3:病因学研究相关性评价

我们能将这个真实的、重要的研究结果应用于我当前的患者吗?	
(1)当前患者是否与病因证据研究对象特征不同?	
(2)该危险因素对当前的患者利弊权衡如何?	
(3)当前患者的偏好、担忧和期望是什么?	

教师:现在时间到了。谁愿意主动把你们的答案写在黑板上,并向我们解释你是如何计算 OR 值的,95%CI 是什么意思?

学生:(写并解释)

教师:OR=71/15÷53/30=2.7,95%CI[1.2,5.8],即高咖啡因摄入者发生尿失禁的概率是不喝咖啡或少量咖啡因摄入者的 2.7 倍。95%: CI[1.2,5.8]表示估计的总体参数有 95% 的可能性落入该区间。而这个可信区间不包含无效值 1,因此具有统计学意义。

请核对你的答案是否和下表一样。

工作表 2:病因学研究重要性评价(核对)

(1)病因与疾病之间的因果相关强度有多大?

(2)暴露与结局之间关联评估的精确性如何?

结局指标

暴　露	逼尿肌不稳定组 （$N=131$）	无副尿肌不稳定组 （$N=128$）	OR	95%CI
咖啡因摄取平均值	484 ± 123 mg/d	194 ± 84 mg/d		
高摄入量 （>100 mg/d）	71(54.2)	53(41.4)	2.7	1.2, 5.8
中等摄入量 （100~400 mg/d）	45(34.4)	45(35.2)	2.0	0.9, 4.5
低摄入量 （<100 mg/d）	15(11.5)	30(23.4)	1.0	

罗希莹

Chapter 7

Critical Appraisal of Risk Factor and Etiological Studies

Part I Teaching Requirements

The first part of this session is an introduction to some concepts of etiology.

The second part of this session is focused on the types of studies and critical appraisal of risk factor and etiological studies, concentrating on reading material and doing some exercises.

1. Teaching aims

To discuss some relevant concepts of etiology, the types of studies and critical appraisal of risk factors and etiology studies.

2. Learning objectives

After completing this session, students should be able to:

(1) Understand some relevant concepts of etiology.

(2) Know the types of etiology study and the inference strength of each.

(3) Critically appraise etiology study.

3. Teaching methods

This session will use lecture, PPT presentation and interactive teaching method. Interactive teaching techniques including think break, wave and appraisal task.

4. Reading materials

(1) Straus S E, Richardson W S, Glasziou P, et al. Evidence-based

medicine：how to practice and teach EBM. 3rd ed. Singapore：Elservier（Singapore）Pte Ltd.，2006.

　　（2）Lily A. Arya，Deborah L. Myers，et al. Dietary caffeine intake and the risk for detrusor instability：a case-control study. Obstetrics & Gynecology，2000，96（1）：85 - 89.

Part II　Teaching Design — 2 periods（80 minutes）

Teaching design of "Critical Appraisal of Risk Factors and Etiological Studies"

No.	Content	Interactive technique/ teaching techniques	Descriptions	Time (minutes)
1	Outline of the course	PPT presentation	Review the three appraisal aspects of therapeutic research，and briefly introduce the content and arrangement of the course in this chapter through PPT.	5
2	Introduction to etiology	PPT presentation Interaction 7.1：Think break	Ask the questions. Let students think about them. Elicit concepts of etiology and risk factors. Introduce the etiology research and its purpose.	5
3	etiology studies, and inference strengh	PPT presentation	Provide students with different types of etiology studies，and analyze inference strength of each.	10
4	Introduction to clinical scenario	PPT presentation Interaction 7.2：TPS	Give students the clinical scenario and reading materials，and ask students to think about how to practice EBM.	10
5	Validity evaluation of etiology study	Interaction 7.3：Wave PPT presentation	Use "wave" to classify students into groups（5 persons/group）. Then，students read Lily A's article，discuss and complete etiology study appraisal worksheet 1.	25
6	Importance and relevance appraisal	Interaction 7.4：Appraisal task	Students complete the appraisal task of importance and relevance of the evidence.	25

Part III   Teaching Contents

1. Outline of the course

The session consists of 3 aspects. They are:
(1) Introduction to Etiology.
(2) Types of etiological studies (case-control studies, cohort studies and randomized controlled trials) and the inference strength of each.
(3) Critical appraisal of etiology study.

2. Introduction to etiology

The teacher asks questions, let student think, elicit concepts of etiology.

Interaction 7.1 : Think break

Teacher: Every day, as medical staff, you may face a variety of questions about disease. In addition to paying attention to the treatment of diseases, you will also frequently be asked "why do I have this disease", "what are the factors which cause my disease". The correct answers to these questions are not only related to clinical decision, but also help effective communication between doctors and patients and their families. In addition, questions about risk factors are often of public concern, such as the following one: does living near hydroelectric lines increase the risk of cancer? If you are asked this question, your answer is?

Student: It doesn't!.

Teacher: Another question: does taking statins for long time cause cancer?

Student: Maybe.

Teacher: Oh, really? Do you have any evidence?

Student: No.

Teacher: Does exposure to aluminum cause Alzheimer's dementia?

Student: Yes.

Teacher: Do you really think so? Why?

Student: I don't know. Maybe ...

Teacher: Does elevated homocysteine level cause coronary artery disease?

Student: I don't know.

Teacher: All these questions are about harm, causes or risks of a disease. To answer these questions, etiological studies are needed, or critical evaluation of the studies that have been done is needed. Let's clarify a few concepts: what is etiological factor, and what is risk factor? What is etiology research and its purpose? I want everybody to think about them, and discuss with your deskmates.

（1）Etiological factors: Refer to the external and objective biological, physical, chemical and social harmful factors, or the adverse psychological state and genetic defects of the human body which will have an effect on the human body under certain conditions and can lead to diseases.

（2）Risk factors: Refer to the factors that have certain cause-effect relationship with the occurrence, development and vanishment of disease, but there is no sufficient evidence to clarify its specific pathogenic effect. However, when these factors exist, the incidence of related diseases (events) will increase correspondingly; when these factors are eliminated, the incidence of the disease decreases. For example, smoking, high blood pressure and hypercholesterolemia are risk factors of ischemic heart disease.

（3）Etiological study: It is a study on the causal relationship between etiological factors or risk factors and diseases. The study on adverse effects caused by interventions is essentially the determination of causation, so also belongs to etiology study.

（4）Etiological study and its purpose

A. To determine causation and estimate the harm.

B. To make intervention decisions (including prevention and treatment) which aim at the causes and risk factors so as to control the disease.

3. Etiological study design and the strength of inference

Ideally, to answer the questions about the cause of diseases, a systematic review or a Meta-analysis that combines all relevant randomized trials or cohort studies might provide us with sufficiently large-scale samples to detect even rare adverse events. Unfortunately, such reviews aren't common, thus the discussion in this chapter will focus on randomized trials, cohort, case-control studies, and descriptive studies.

Etiology research methods are ranked according to the strength of causal inference: systematic review, single randomized controlled trial, cohort study, case-control study, and descriptive study, as shown in the following table.

Strength of inference in etiological studies

Design	Starting point	Outcome	Advantage	Disadvantage	Inference strength
RCT	exposure	adverse event	prospective, good comparability	ethical issue, pool feasibility	++++
cohort study	exposure	adverse event	prospective, comparision	non-randomization confunding	+++
case-control study	adverse event	exposure	small sample size, no ethical issue	recall bias confunding	++
descriptive study	exposure	adverse event	simple, good feasibility	no comparision	+

（1）Randomized controlled trials: In randomized controlled trials, subjects were randomly assigned into the experimental group and control group. One of the reasons for the strong strength of inference is that random allocation can evenly distribute factors (known and unknown) that may affect outcome among groups, thus eliminating the influence of unknown confoundings, and the researcher can actively control the exposure factors or treatment measures.

However, two factors limit the use of randomized controlled trials to study the pathogenic effects of adverse reactions or exposure factors. On one hand, when we suspect that an intervention or exposure factor may be harmful, there are ethical issues in randomly assigning subjects to the experimental group and the control group to accept the factors that may be harmful to them. On the other hand, when rare, severe, adverse reactions of interventions with long incubation period are studied, a large sample size and long period of observation are required, which is less feasible.

(2) Cohort study: According to whether some exposure factors are contacted or not, observed population is naturally divided into two groups and after following up for a period of time, researchers compare the difference of the occurrence of a certain disease between the groups. The difference between cohort studies and randomized controlled trials is that the exposure of the observed subjects is not randomly assigned, but is determined by the observed population or is formed naturally. Cohort studies are susceptible to confoundings due to the fact that exposure factors naturally exist in the population and researchers cannot actively control them.

(3)Case-control study: It is a retrospective study method. For cases with adverse reactions and cases without adverse reactions, it retrospectively investigates the conditions of contacting a certain intervention or exposure factor, and compares the two groups. It is suitable for the study of rare and long incubation period diseases. It takes less time, less costs and less effort, and harmless to patients, so has no ethical issues. Meanwhile, it can explore the possible relationship between multiple exposures and study outcomes. However, because the information is completely based on recalling, it is easy to produce recalling bias. It is also more susceptible to confoundings. Therefore, case-control study can only deduce the possible causal relationship, but cannot verify the causation.

4. A clinical scenario

Introduce a clinical scenario and ask students to think about how to practice EBM.

Interaction 7.2 : TPS

Teacher: Suppose you were a clinician. One day, a patient came to the clinic. The following was her situation: A 45-year-old woman complained of urge incontinence which had gotten progressively worse over the last 2 years, significantly impacting her quality of life. Her past history was remarkable for three pregnancies (the reason why she had urge urinary incontinence is associated with each of these), and forceps were used during two of the births. She took lorazepam occasionally at night for difficult sleeping. She was on no other medications and had no smoking history. Her caffeine intake consisted of 750mL (25 oz) of coffee per day. Her clinical examination was unremarkable except for visible urine leakage when she was asked to cough while in the lithotomy position. Her post-void residual urine volume was 20 mL and a urinalysis was unremarkable. She recently read in the paper that caffeine can cause urinary incontinence and wanted to know if this is true or if there are other factors that could be contributing to her problem.

Who can answer the patient's question? If you can't, what should you do? Can you tell me the steps to practice EBM?

Student 1: Ask questions, find evidence, evaluate evidence, apply evidence, and do after-effect evaluation.

Teacher: Very good! Let's start with the first step and ask clinical questions. Do you still remember the structure of the clinical problems?

Student 2: PICO.

Teacher: The patient wants to know if coffee taking can cause urinary incontinence, or make it worse. This is a question about etiology, so the structure of the question should be modified to PECO; E means the exposure factor. Now, I will ask two students to write their clinical questions on the blackboard.

Student 3: For a 45-year-old woman, does coffee cause urinary incontinence?

Student 4: For women with urinary incontinence, does 750 milliliters of coffee per day increase the risk of urinary incontinence?

Teacher: Ok, we got two questions now. Which do you think is better? Second, yes, P is for women with urinary incontinence, E is for coffee or caffeine intake (excessive dietary caffeine intake), and C is for those who do not, or consume less. O is incontinence or incontinence getting worse. Now let's move on to the second step, search for the evidence. We can use "urge incontinence AND (coffee OR caffeine)"to search for different levels of evidence. What is the highest level of evidence for etiology?

Student: Systematic review or Meta-analysis.

Teacher: Right! Now if we get the following four articles, please rank them according to the levels of evidence. Please think and discuss with your deskmates. After 5 minutes, I will ask some of you to write down their answers on the blackboard.

(1) Coffee and caffeine intake and risk of urinary incontinence: a Meta-analysis of observational studies.

(2) Prevalence and risk factors for urinary incontinence in Italy: a cross-sectional study.

(3) Prevalence and risk factors for urine leakage in a racially and ethnically diverse population of adults: a cohort study.

(4) Is caffeine intake associated with urinary incontinence in Japanese adults: a case-control study.

The rank according to the level of the evidence is just the same rank as the causal inference strength of the etiological study design. That is, a systematic review/Meta-analysis that combines all relevant randomized trials or cohort studies might provide us with sufficient large number of patients to detect even rare advance events ranks at the top. Etiological studies are usually unable to design RCTs due to ethical limitations. Therefore, large sample observational studies, such as cohort studies, are the highest level of original research evidence; then there are case control studies and descriptive studies. Did you get the order right?

5. Validity appraisal of etiological study

Introduce validity worksheet to students. Ask them to read Lily A's literature, complete the worksheet, discuss with deskmates and share with the class.

Interaction 7.3：Wave

Students read the assigned article, discuss it within the group, and complete valitity appraisal.

Teacher: Let's do a wave activity. Now I need you to call out a number from 1 to 5 one by one. (5 persons per group, if needed, 4 persons per group, call out 1 to 4, and so on; the number of class students is assumed as 50.) Please be sure to remember the number of yourself.

Students: (call out the numbers)

Teacher: Ok, all number 1 students stand up please, sit down please. All number 2, sit down please. number 3, and 4, and 5. Great! Now I want the first number, that is all number 1 of course, stand up and raise you arms and call out your number in the meantime, and sit down before the next number stand up, number by number as one falls another rises.

Students: (do the wave)

Teacher: We have 5 groups now. The same number will be in the same group. Every group please find a table, and sit down, then read the following paper and discuss the validity of the study, and complete the worksheet 1.

Lily A. Arya, Deborah L. Myers et al. Dietary caffeine intake and the risk for detrusor instability: a case-control study. Obstetrics & Gynecology, 2000, 96(1): 85 – 89.

Students: (read and discus)

Worksheet 1: Validity appraisal of etiological study

Is this evidence about etiology valid?	Yes/No/ Not clear	Citation expression in the article
(1) Was the etiological evidence based on a strong inference study design?		
(2) Were treatments/exposures and clinical outcomes measured in the same way in both groups? (Was the assessment of outcomes either objective or blinded to exposure?)		
(3) Was the follow-up of the patients in the study sufficiently long (for the outcome to occur) and complete?		

(continued)

Is this evidence about etiology valid?	Yes/No/ Not clear	Citation expression in the article
(4) Do the results of the etiological study satisfy some of the diagnostic tests for causation? — Is it clear that the exposure preceded the onset of the outcome? — Is there a dose-response gradient? — Is there any positive evidence from a "dechallenge-rechallenge" study — Is the association consistent from study to study? — Does the association make biological sense?		

Teacher：Ok，let's check your worksheet.

（1）Was the etiological evidence based on a strong inference study design?

The article is a case-control study which has moderate inference strengh.

（2）Were treatments/exposures and clinical outcomes measured in the same way in both groups?

Participants in both the control and the case group were asked to complete a 48-hour voiding diary before urodynamic testing.

This diary consisted of a structured intake and output diary to record the type and amount of fluid. They were asked to record their intake of coffee，tea，cola，and cocoa using a measuring cup. The reproducibility of this diary was assessed in a random sample of women after an interval of 1 week. It does not state if the patients were aware of the study hypothesis. Medical charts were reviewed to obtain information about potential confounders，including parity and smoking history.

（3）Was the follow-up of the patients in the study sufficiently long （for the outcome to occur）and complete?

The study population consisted of 259 consecutive women who were evaluated for urinary incontinence at our tertiary referral urodynamic center between October 1996 and July 1998.

Women were asked to record their intake of coffee（caffeinated or decaffeinated, instant or brewed), tea, cola (with brand name), and cocoa using a measuring cup. The reproducibility of this diary in assessing caffeine intake was examined by retesting, after an interval of 1 week. All subjects were taken into final statistical analysis in their initially assigned group.

(4) Do the results of the harm study satisfy some of the diagnostic tests for causation?

Because this is a retrospective case-control study, causal sequence is not clear, which needs more evidence.

6. Importance and relevance appraisal

(1) Are the valid results of this etiological study important?

A. What is the magnitude of the association between the exposure and outcome?

B. What is the precision of the estimate of the association between the exposure and outcome?

(2) Can this valid and important evidence about harm be applied to our patient?

A. Is our patient so different from those included in the study?

B. What are our patient's benefit and harm from this exposure?

C. What are our patient's preferences, concerns, and expectations?

D. Is there any other alternative therapy?

Interaction 7.4 : Task

Teacher: (distribute etiology study appraisal worksheet 2 and worksheet 3) Please fill in the two worksheets based on:

Lily A. Arya, Deborah L. Myers, et al. Dietary caffeine intake and the risk for detrusor instability: a case-control study. Obstetrics & Gynecology, 2000, 96(1): 85 - 89.

Then discuss it with your deskmates. We have 25 minutes.

Students: (practice and discus)

Worksheet 2: Importance appraisal of etiological study

(1) What is the magnitude of the association between the exposure and outcome?

(2) What is the precision of the estimate of the association between the exposure and outcome?

Outcomes according to study group:

exposure	Detrusor instability group ($N=$　)	No detrusor instability group ($N=$　)	OR	95%CI
Mean caffeine intake				
High ($>$100 mg/d)				
Moderate (100 – 400 mg/d)				
Minimal ($<$100 mg/d)				

Worksheet 3: Relevance appraisal of etiological study

Can we apply this valid, important evidence about etiology to our patient?	
(1) Is our patient so different from those included in the study?	
(2) What are our patient's benefit and harm from this exposure?	
(3) What are our patient's preferences, concerns, and expectations?	

Teacher: Now, time is up. I would like to ask some volunteers to write their answers on the blackboard and explain to us how you calculated OR, and what the 95% CI means?

Student: (write and explain)

Teacher: $OR = 71/15 \div 53/30 = 2.7$, 95% CI[1.2, 5.8], means high caffeine intaker was 2.7 times more likely to develop urinary incontinence than non-coffee intaker or minimal caffeine intaker. 95% CI[1.2, 5.8] means that there is a 95% chance that the estimated population parameter falls in the interval, and this confidence interval does not include invalid value 1, so there is statistical significance.

Please check whether your answers are the same as the following worksheet.

Worksheet 2: Importance appraisal of etiology study (check)

(1) What is the magnitude of the association between the exposure and outcome?

(2) What is the precision of the estimate of the association between the exposure and outcome?

Outcomes according to study group:

Exposure	Detrusor instability group ($N=131$)	No detrusor instability group ($N=128$)	OR	95%CI
Mean caffeine intake	484 ± 123 mg/d	194 ± 84 mg/d		
High ($>$100 mg/d)	71(54.2)	53(41.4)	2.7	1.2, 5.8
Moderate (100 – 400 mg/d)	45(34.4)	45(35.2)	2.0	0.9, 4.5
Minimal ($<$100 mg/d)	15(11.5)	30(23.4)	1.0	

Luo Xiying

第 8 章

诊断性研究的严格评价

第一部分　教　学　要　求

诊断性试验可以是有助于诊断疾病的任何试验和方法,包括询问病史、体格检查、实验室或者影像诊断,以及各种诊断标准。此教学环节主要介绍诊断性研究的严格评价,以及如何通过诊断试验重新估计患病概率。

1. 教学目的

学生通过应用诊断试验证据提高对疾病的诊断水平,具体包括:
(1) 诊断试验研究。
(2) 诊断试验研究的要素。
(3) 诊断试验研究的指标。
(4) 诊断试验研究的评价。

2. 学习目标

通过此环节的学习,学生能够:
(1) 给诊断试验下定义。
(2) 列出诊断试验研究的要素。
(3) 计算诊断试验所涉及的一些性能指标,如灵敏度、特异度、预测值和似然比。
(4) 了解验前概率和验后概率,以及如何在临床实践中进行推导;了解在给定的验前概率和似然比下,如何应用列线图确定疾病的验后概率。
(5) 能够进行诊断性研究的真实性、重要性和相关性评价。

3. 教学方法

此环节采用讲授法、PPT 演示和互动教学法,互动教学技术包括教师讲故事、TPS。

4. 阅读材料

Arnedos M，Nerurkar A，Osin P，et al. Discordance between core needle biopsy（CNB）and excisional biopsy（EB）for estrogen receptor（ER），progesterone receptor（PgR）and HER2 status in early breast cancer（EBC）．Annals of Oncology Official Journal of the European Society for Medical Oncology，2009，20(12)：1948.

第二部分　教学设计——2 课时（80 分钟）

"诊断性研究的严格评价"教学设计表

序号	内　容	互动技术/教学技术	描　　　　述	时间（分钟）
1	诊断性试验简介	互动 8.1：教师讲故事 PPT 演示	教师通过真实案例,让学生思考故事中患者出现症状和体征的可能原因,以及将如何诊断该患者,引出：① 诊断试验的定义；② 诊断性试验研究；③ 诊断性试验研究的目的	10
2	诊断性试验研究的要素	PPT 演示	介绍诊断性试验研究的要素：① 采用标准诊断（或金标准）；② 新的诊断试验；③ 研究对象；④ 盲法比较	10
3	诊断性试验研究的指标	PPT 演示	诊断性试验研究的指标及四格表：① 灵敏度（SEN）；② 特异度（SPE）；③ 阳性预测值（PV ＋）；④ 似然比（LR）；⑤ 阳性似然比（LR＋）	20
4	诊断指标的意义	PPT 演示	用 SEN、SPE、PV 等诊断指标解释试验结果	10
5	诊断性试验研究的评价	PPT 演示	介绍诊断性试验研究评价的三个方面	10
6	诊断试验研究的真实性、重要性、相关性评价任务	互动 8.2：TPS	请学生回忆循证医学实践的步骤,阅读 Arnedos M 的文献,并完成工作表 1～3,配对讨论并在全班分享	20

第三部分　教　学　内　容

1. 诊断性试验简介

　　早期、正确地诊断疾病是实施适当治疗和估计预后的基础。然而,大多数情况的诊断和治疗都需要复杂的步骤和周密的考虑。临床医师将收集包括病史、症状、体格检查、实验室检测、影像检查,甚至一些特殊检查等信息,并对所有的信息和数据进行全面分析,以进行诊断。诊断过程是一种直觉和推理的整合。

　　一个好的医生会根据他们的医学素养和经验来诊断,但是真正的临床情况要复杂得多,你需要练习循证医学技术来支持诊断决策,也即根据临床问题找到诊断证据,并对证据进行评估,然后应用证据进行诊断决策。

　　本章课程将重点讨论诊断性测试,如何评估诊断研究以及如何将其应用于临床情况。

　　以下是一个案例。

互动 8.1：教师讲故事

　　教师：我的一个女性朋友,今年 48 岁,是两个孩子的母亲。近日,她发现自己一侧乳房有包块,因此向外科医生咨询此事。

　　如果你是这个外科医生,请思考导致她的症状和体征可能的病因,并且设想你将如何进行诊断。

　　学生 1：肿块可能是乳腺癌。

　　学生 2：也可能是乳腺炎或者是一个良性的肿瘤。

　　教师：嗯,那你们将怎么来诊断呢?

　　学生 3：让她做一个超声检查。

　　教师：超声检查,嗯,还有吗?

　　学生 4：X 线检查。

　　教师：很好！但是否有哪个同学认为首先询问病史及为患者进行体检比一来就让患者去做诊断测试,如超声检查或 X 线检查更重要呢?

　　学生：哦,是这样。

　　教师：是的,你们首先要做的是问清病史,为患者做体检。事实上,诊断试验其实包括了所有获得有助于明确病症的信息的方法,包括询问病史、体格检查。当然,诊断试验多指医院内开展的实验室诊断和影像学诊断。

　　下面,我们来学习诊断试验的定义。

（1）诊断试验：是用于诊断或发现疾病、损伤或其他医学异常情况的实验和方法。

（2）诊断试验研究：对一种新的诊断试验灵敏度、特异度等方面进行的研究。

（3）诊断试验研究的重要性/目的：诊断是疾病治疗的先决条件。原有的诊断方法（即使是金标准）有些可能是有创的，如有创性的冠状动脉造影诊断心肌梗死；有些可能费用较高，如 PET CT 诊断肿瘤；有些可能耗时较长，如 DNA 检测诊断 AIDS 和两性畸形等。而诊断试验研究的目的就是发现更少损伤、更少花费、更省时又更有效的方法，从而修正疾病存在或不存在的可能性。

2. 诊断试验研究的要素

（1）使用标准诊断（金标准）："金标准"是迄今公认诊断某种疾病最准确和最可靠的方法，不仅能准确地确诊目标疾病，还能排除相似的其他疾病，如组织活检、尸检、手术发现、细菌培养、病原体分离。然而，很多疾病还没有任何的金标准，而且有些金标准是非常昂贵的和耗时的，也有损伤。

在一个诊断试验研究中，金标准和新的诊断试验应该进行盲法、独立的同步比较。

（2）新的诊断试验：欲进行研究的一种新的诊断方法。常常是更少损伤、更少花费，或更快的方法。

（3）研究对象：诊断试验所研究的患者样本应该纳入临床实践中将使用该诊断试验的各种患者类型，即研究的样本中应当既有目标疾病较轻微的病例，又有严重的病例；既有早期病例又有晚期病例；并且将经过治疗和未经过治疗的个体都包括在内。

（4）盲法比较：进行诊断性研究时，应用盲法对比诊断性试验结果和金标准诊断结果，即诊断性试验的实施、结果判断不能受金标准的影响，反之亦然。此外，诊断性试验和金标准试验最好同步进行，其间隔时间不能太长，以免病情变化影响结果的准确性。

3. 诊断性试验研究的指标和四格表

在循证医学实践中常用的诊断试验评价指标包括灵敏度（SEN）、特异度（SPE）、阳性预测值（PV＋）、阳性似然比（LR＋）等。通常我们使用四格表来呈现测试的结果，并计算以上指标值。

诊断试验四格表

新的诊断试验	金　标　准		合　计
	有病	无病	
阳性＋	a（真阳＋）	b（假阳＋）	a＋b
阴性－	c（假阴－）	d（真阴－）	a＋c
合　计	a＋c	b＋d	N＝a＋b＋c＋d

（1）灵敏度（SEN）：有病者诊断试验阳性的比例，SEN＝a/(a＋c)。

（2）特异度（SPE）：无病者诊断试验阴性的比例，SPE＝d/(b＋d)。

（3）准确度（ACC）：诊断性试验正确诊断的比例，ACC＝(a＋d)/N。

（4）阳性预测值（PV＋）：诊断性试验阳性者中患病者的比例，PV＋＝a/(a＋b)。

（5）似然比（LR）：阳性或阴性的测试结果在多大程度上改变了患病的概率，并以比率表示。

（6）阳性似然比（LR＋）：有病者诊断性试验阳性的概率和无病者诊断试验阳性的概率之比，可用灵敏度和特异度表达，LR＋＝[a/(a＋c)]/[b/(b＋d)]＝SEN/(1－SPE)。

似然比为0到无穷大：LR＝0，说明诊断试验没有提供额外的信息；LR＞1，患病的可能性增加；LR＜1，患病的可能性降低。

4. 应用 SEN、SPE、PV 解释诊断试验的结果

灵敏度和特异度可以用于以下情况：

（1）灵敏度高的诊断试验，当试验结果为阴性时，可以排除疾病。

（2）特异度高的诊断试验，当试验结果为阳性时，可以判断有病。

疾病预测值由灵敏度和特异度决定，但也受受试人群的患病率影响。因此，预测值在帮助医生确定特定人群的患病概率时，其作用是有限的。不同人群常常有不同的验前概率。

诊断试验的重要性在于能否明显改变验前医生对患者患病概率（验前概率）的估计，得到诊断试验结果后，医生应根据诊断试验结果重新估计患者患病的概率（验后概率）：

验前概率＋试验信息（似然比）＝验后概率

能否从验前概率估计验后概率，取决于诊断试验的似然比。

假设某患者的验前概率是30%，LR＋＝1.71：

验前比＝验前概率/(1－验前概率)＝0.3/(1－0.3)＝0.43

验后比＝验前比 * 似然比＝0.43 * 1.71＝0.73

验后概率＝验后比/(1＋验后比)＝0.73/(1＋0.73)＝42%

使用似然比运算图可以方便地直接从验前概率(30%)和阳性似然比(1.7)直接获得验后概率。在左侧的标尺上找到验前概率(30%),中间标尺上找到似然比(1.71),以直线连接两点并延伸至与右侧标尺相交,交点刻度即为验后概率(42%)。

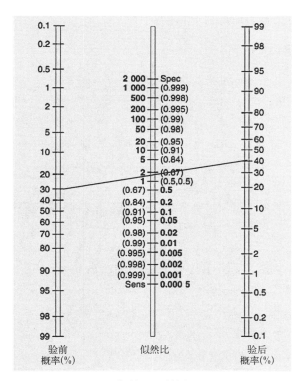

似然比运算图

5. 诊断性试验研究的评价

(1)真实性评价

A. 是否包括适当的疾病谱? 研究对象应与临床实际情况相似,纳入所有可能与所研究疾病混淆的对象,以及疾病的各种类型和不同时期。

B. 是否采用了金标准进行比较? 标准诊断(或金标准)指的是目前公认的确诊目标疾病的诊断方法。

C. 是否与金标准进行了盲法比较？为避免潜在的偏倚,判断诊断试验结果者不能预告知道其他诊断的结果。

（2）重要性评价

A. 诊断试验的结果是什么？

B. 试验结果是否呈现似然比,以及计算似然比所必需的数据？

（3）适用性评价（或关联性）

A. 测试结果的可重复性及其解释的是否令人满意？

B. 结果是否适用于我的患者？

C. 测试的结果是否对患者有帮助？

6. 评价任务（真实性评价）

互动 8.2：TPS

教师：大家是否还记得我的朋友：

（1）48 岁的女性,因单侧乳房肿块向医生咨询。

（2）她是两个孩子的母亲。

（3）如果你是一名外科医生。

（4）你询问了她的病史,并实施了体检,然后为她预约了超声诊断。

（5）超声诊断提示恶性肿瘤可能。

（6）你建议她做一个 CNB（芯针活组织检查）以确定治疗策略。

（7）患者的问题是：CNB 是否与 EB（切取活检）的诊断效果一样（能否确定类型和分级等）？

各位同学请根据上面所提供的临床资料,完成以下任务：

（1）提出一个可回答的临床问题。

（2）查找证据（此步省略）。

（3）请阅读下面这篇文献并与同伴讨论：

Arnedos M, Nerurkar A, Osin P, et al. Discordance between core needle biopsy（CNB）and excisional biopsy（EB）for estrogen receptor（ER）, progesterone receptor（PgR）and HER2 status in early breast cancer（EBC）. Annals of Oncology Official Journal of the European Society for Medical Oncology, 2009, 20(12)：1948.

（4）填写工作表 1～3。

学生：（独立思考,与同伴讨论并在全班分享）

（1）诊断性试验研究的真实性评价。

工作表 1：诊断性试验研究的真实性评价

结　果　真　实　性	是	否	不清楚
1. 是否与金标准进行了独立、盲法比较？			
2. 诊断试验是否包括了合适的疾病谱？			
3. 不管诊断试验结果如何，是否都采用了金标准进行诊断？			
4. 诊断试验是否提供了足够的细节以供复制？			

（2）诊断性试验研究的重要性评价：计算灵敏度、特异度、阳性似然比和准确度。

工作表 2：诊断性试验研究的重要性评价

试验结果是什么(结果是否重要?)			
EB			
CNB	＋	－	合　计
ER＋			
ER－			
合　计			
SEN			
SPE			
LR＋			
ACC			

基于 Arnedos M 文献中的诊断试验四格表，计算灵敏度、特异度、阳性似然比和准确度如下。

基于 Arnedos M 文献的诊断试验四格表

CNB	EB		合　计
	＋	－	
ER＋	251	2	253
ER－	4	79	83
合　计	255	81	336

通过计算,SEN=98.4,SPE=97.5,ACC=98,LR+=39.36。

(3)诊断性试验研究证据的相关性(或适用性)评价及验后概率的计算与意义。

工作表 3:诊断性试验研究的适用性评价

该试验结果可以应用于我当前的患者吗?	
该诊断方法在本地可获得否? 患者能否支付? 准确性如何?	
你能否准确地估计你当前患者的验前概率?	
验后概率是否有助于你治疗当前患者?	
测试结果是否对患者有所帮助?	

假设,验前概率(或称患病率)为 60%,则:

验前比＝验前概率/(1－验前概率)＝0.6/(1－0.6)＝1.5

验后比＝验前比 * 似然比＝1.5×39.36＝59.04

验后概率＝验后比/(1＋验后比)＝59.04/(1＋59.04)＝0.98

验后概率意味着在该试验的患病率(60%)情况下,患者若获得 CNB 阳性结果,则有 98%的把握诊断该病。

验后概率也可通过似然比运算图获得。

李红梅

Chapter 8

Critical Appraisal of Diagnostic Studies

Part I   Teaching Requirements

Diagnostic tests may include any type of test or method that could be helpful in making a diagnosis, including history-taking and physical examination, laboratory or imaging test, and various diagnostic reference standard. This session is about how to appraise diagnostic research critically and how to use diagnostic test to refine the probability of diseases.

1. Teaching aims

To show students how to improve the use of diagnostic tests by learning to apply the evidence-based techniques of refining the probability of disease. It includes:

(1) Diagnostic test study.

(2) Elements for diagnostic test study.

(3) Indicators for diagnostic test study.

(4) Appraisal of diagnostic test study.

2. Learning objectives

After completing this session, students should be able to:

(1) Define the diagnostic test.

(2) List the elements for diagnostic test study.

(3) Calculate some parameters involved in diagnostic test, such as specificity, predictive values and likelihood ratios.

(4) Understand the concepts of pre-test and post-test probability of diseases and how they are derived in clinical practice. Understand and use a

nomogram to define post-test probability of disease，with given indicators of pre-test probability and likelihood ratio.

（5）Critically evaluate validity，importance and relevance of diagnostic studies.

3. Teaching methods

This session will use lecture，PPT presentation and interactive teaching method. Interactive teaching techniques include instructor storytelling and TPS.

4. Reading materials

Arnedos M，Nerurkar A，Osin P，et al. Discordance between core needle biopsy（CNB）and excisional biopsy（EB）for estrogen receptor（ER），progesterone receptor（PgR）and HER2 status in early breast cancer（EBC）. Annals of Oncology Official Journal of the European Society for Medical Oncology，2009，20（12）：1948.

Part II Teaching Design — 2 periods（80 minutes）

Teaching design of "Critical Appraisal of Diagnostic Studies"

No.	Content	Interactive technique/ teaching techniques	Descriptions	Time（minutes）
1	Introduction to diagnostic test	Interaction 8.1： Instructor storytelling PPT presentation	Teacher illustrates a story of a real case，asking students to think about what are the possible cause of the symptom and sign，and how you would diagnose the problem. Elicit：① the definition of diagnostic test；② diagnostic test study；③ the purpose of a diagnostic test study.	10
2	Elements for diagnostic test study	PPT presentation	Introduce the elements for diagnostic test study：① use of reference standard（Gold Standard）；② new diagnostic test；③ subjects；④ comparison with blind method.	10

（continued）

No.	Content	Interactive technique/ teaching techniques	Descriptions	Time (minutes)
3	Indicators for diagnostic test study	PPT presentation	Indicators for diagnostic test study and the 2×2 table (fourfold table): ① sensitivity; ② specificity; ③ positive predictive value; ④ likelihood ratio; ⑤ positive likelihood ratio.	20
4	Interpreting test results	PPT presentation	Interpreting test results using SEN, SPE, PV.	10
5	Appraisal of diagnostic test study	PPT presentation	Introduce 3 aspects of the critical appraisal of diagnostic test study.	10
6	Appraising task-validity, importance and relevance appraisal	Interaction 8.2: TPS	Ask student to review the steps of practicing EBM, and read the paper by Arnedos M, fill the worksheet1 – 3, then discuss in pair, and share in the class.	20

Part III Teaching Contents

1. Introduction to diagnostic test

An early correct diagnosis of disease serves as a foundation of implementing proper treatment and evaluating prognosis. In most cases, however, diagnosis and treatment require complex steps and careful considerations. The clinicians will collect information including medical history, symptoms and signs, laboratory tests, image data and even some special examinations, and analyze all the information and data comprehensively to make the diagnosis. Diagnostic process is always a integration of intuition and inference.

A good doctor would follow intuitions based on their medical expertise and experience to diagnose firstly, but real clinical situation is more complex. You need to practice EBM techniques to get the support. That is to find diagnostic evidence based on the clinical question and appraise the evidence, and then apply the evidence to the diagnostic decision.

In this session, we will focus on the diagnostic test, how to evaluate diagnostic research and how to apply them to clinical situation.

Interaction 8.1 : Instructor storytelling

Teacher: A friend of mine is a 48-year-old female. She is a mother of two children. Recently, she consulted a general surgeon for having a mass of unilateral breast.

If you were this surgeon, please think about what the possible causes of the symptom and sign are, and how you would diagnose.

Student 1: The mass could be a breast cancer.

Student 2: Could be mastitis or a benign neoplasms.

Teacher: Ok, how would you diagnose the problem?

Student 3: Perform ultrasound.

Teacher: Ultrasound! Ok! Anything else?

Student 4: X-ray?

Teacher: Good! Is there anyone who thinks it is the most important to take medical history and give the patient a physical examination first, rather than order a diagnostic test, such as ultrasound or X-ray?

Students: Oh, Yes!

Teacher: Yes! You should take the patient's history and give her a physical examination first. Actually, diagnostic test may include any type of information that could be helpful in making a diagnosis, including history-taking and physical examination, but the term is usually applied to a ward, laboratory or imaging tests.

Below is the definition of diagnostic test.

---

(1) Diagnostic test: It is the test or method which is performed to aid in the diagnosis or detection of diseases, injuries or any other medical condition.

(2) Diagnostic test study: Study on new diagnostic tests for their sensitivity, specificity, etc.

（3）Importance/purposes of diagnostic test study: Diagnosis is the preconditions for therapies. But the original diagnostic method（even gold standard）may be invasive, like Invasive Coronary Angiography for myocardial infarction; may be costly, like Pet-CT for cancer; may be time-consuming, like DNA test for AIDS and hermaphrodism etc. The goal of diagnostic testing research is to find less invasive, less costly, less time-consuming, and more effective ways to refine the possibility that the disease may or may not exist.

2. Elements for diagnostic test study

（1）The use of reference standard（Gold Standard）: Gold Standard is the current recognized best available diagnostic test for a target disorder, with which, target disease can be confirmed accurately, and similar other diseases can be ruled out, such as biopsy, autopsy, surgical findings, bacterial culture, pathogens isolation. However, there have been no "gold standard" to many diseases, and some of the gold standards are costly, time-consuming, and invasive as above mentioned.

In a diagnostic test study, both gold standard and new diagnostic test should be applied to the patient samples independently, blindly.

（2）New diagnostic test: A new diagnostic approach to be studied, often one that is less invasive, less costly, or faster.

（3）Subjects: The patient sample should include an appropriate spectrum of patients to whom the diagnostic tests will be applied in clinical practice. Actually, the really useful study will be set in the diagnostic dilemmas we face, and include patients with mild as well as severe symptoms, early as well as late cases of the target disorder, and among both treated and untreated individuals.

（4）Comparison with blind method: When conducting diagnostic test study, the results of diagnostic test should be compared with those of gold standard blindly, that is, the implementation and result judgment of diagnostic tests should not be affected by gold standard, and vice versa. In addition, the diagnostic test and the gold standard test should be carried out synchronously, and the interval should not be too long, so as to avoid the change of the condition affecting the accuracy of the results.

3. Indicators for diagnostic test study and the fourfold table

The common evaluative indicators for diagnostic tests used in EMB include sensitivity（SEN），specificity（SPE），positive predictive value（PV+），and positive likelihood ratio（LR+），etc.

We use a fourfold table to present test outcomes，and calculate the following indicators.

Diagnostic test fourfold table

New diagnostic test	Gold standard		Total
	Presence	Absence	
Test positive +	a（true+）	b（false+）	a+b
Test negative−	c（false−）	d（true −）	a+c
Total	a+c	b+d	N=a+b+c+d

（1）Sensitivity（SEN）：probability of a positive test when disease is present，SEN=a/(a+c).

（2）Specificity（SPE）：probability of a negative test when disease is absent，SPE=d/(b+d).

（3）Accuracy（ACC）：probability of correct diagnosis，ACC=(a+d)/N.

（4）Positive predictive value（PV+）：probability of disease in patients with a positive test result，PV+=a/(a+b).

（5）likelihood ratio：defines how much a positive or negative test result modifies the probability of disease，and is expressed as a ratio.

（6）Positive likelihood ratio（LR+）：The ratio of probability of a positive test result in patients with the disease to probability of a positive test result in patients without the disease. Likelihood ratio can be defined in terms of sensitivity and specificity.

$$LR+=[a/(a+c)]/[b/(b+d)]=SEN/(1-SPE)$$

LR ranges from 0 to infinity. LR = 0，means the test provides no additional information；LR>1，increases the likelihood of disease；LR<1，decreases the likelihood of disease.

4. Interpreting test results using SEN, SPE, PV

Sensitivity and specificity are occasionally helpful:

(1) A highly sensitive test, when negative, rules out disease (SenOut).

(2) A highly specific test, when positive, rules in disease (SpeIn).

The predictive value is determined by the sensitivity and specificity of the test, but also by the prevalence of disease in the population being tested. Predictive value may therefore be of limited value in helping us refine probability in our particular patient population, which usually has a different prevalence/pretest probability of disease.

The importance of the diagnostic test is whether it can significantly change in estimate of the patient's probability of disease (pre-test probability). After we get the results of the diagnostic test, we should refine the patient's probability of disease (post-test probability) based on the results of the diagnostic test.

Pre-test probability +test information (likelihood ratio)=post-test probability

Moving from an initial assessment of the likelihood of disease (pre-test probability), to determine a final assessment of disease likelihood (post-test probability).

Likelihood ratios are an alternate method of assessing the performance of a diagnostic test.

Given that a patient is with pre-test probability=30%, LR+=1.71:

Pre-test odds =pretest probability/(1−pre-test probability)

$$=0.3/(1-0.3)=0.43$$

Post-test odds=pre-test odds×LR+=0.43×1.71=0.73

Post-test probability =post-test odds/(1+ Post-test odds)

$$=0.73/(1+0.73)=42\%$$

Using the following nomogram, you can easily determine the post-test probability of disease for this patent with a 30% pre-test probability and LR+=1.7. Find the pre-test probability (30%) on the left scale and the likelihood ratio (1.71) on the middle scale. Connect the two points and extend the line to the right scale to intersect. The intersection point on the scale is the post-test probability (42%).

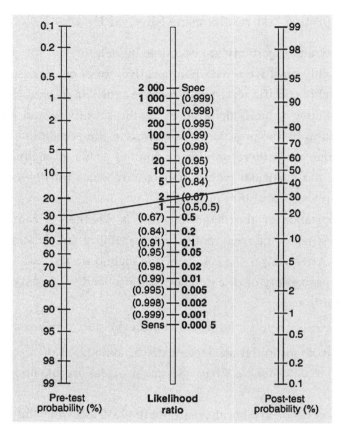

Likelihood ratio nomogram

5. Appraisal of evidence on diagnostic test study

（1）Validity

A. Spectrum of disease? The subjects selected should be similar to the clinical situation，including all subjects that may be confused with the target disease and different periods of different types of the disease.

B. Is the test compared with reference/gold standard? The reference/gold standard refers to the commonly accepted proof that the target disorder is present or not.

C. Did researchers conduct the test blind to the reference standard? To avoid potential bias，those conducting the test should not know or be aware of the results of the other test.

(2) Importance

A. What were the results?

B. Are likelihood ratios for the test results presented or data necessary for their calculation provided?

(3) Relevance (or applicability)

A. Will the reproducibility of the test results and their interpretation be satisfactory in my setting?

B. Are the results applicable to my patient?

C. Will patients be better off as a result of the test?

6. Appraisal task(validity appraisal)

Interaction 8.2 : TPS

Teacher: Do you still remember the friend of mine?

(1) A 48-year-old female patient with a mass of unilateral breast consults you.

(2) She is a mother of two children.

(3) You are a general surgeon.

(4) You gather her medical history, give her a physical examination and order an ultrosonography.

(5) Ultrosonography indicates malignancy.

(6) You suggest CNB (core needle biopsy) to determine treatment strategy.

(7) Patient's question: Is CNB the same as EB (excisional biopsy) in confirming diagnosis (type, grade, etc.)?

According to above clinical scenario, complete the following tasks:

(1) Ask an answerable clinical question.

(2) Searching for evidence (omit this step).

(3) Reading this article and discuss it in pairs:

Arnedos M, Nerurkar A, Osin P, et al. Discordance between core needle biopsy (CNB) and excisional biopsy (EB) for estrogen receptor (ER), progesterone receptor (PgR) and HER2 status in early breast cancer (EBC). Annals of Oncology Official Journal of the European Society for Medical Oncology, 2009, 20(12): 1948.

（4）Complete the diagnostic Worksheet 1 - 3.

Students：（think individually，discuss the result in pairs and share it in public）

（1）Validity appraisal of diagnostic test study

Worksheet 1：Validity appraisal of diagnostic test study

Are the results of the study valid?	Yes	No	Not clear
1. Was there an independent，blind comparison with a reference（gold）standard of diagnosis?			
2. Was the diagnostic test evaluated in an appropriate spectrum of patients?			
3. Was the reference（gold）standard applied regardless of the diagnostic test result?			
4. Were the methods for performing the test described in sufficient detail to permit replication?			

（2）Importance appraisal of diagnostic test study：Calculate SEN，SPE，LR+and ACC.

Worksheet 2：Importance appraisal of diagnostic test study

What are the results?（Is the result important?）			
EB			
CNB	+	—	TOTAL
ER+			
ER−			
TOTAL			
SEN			
SPE			
LR+			
ACC			

SEN，SPE，LR+ and ACC based on the diagnostic test fourfold table in Arnedos M's paper are calculated as follows.

Diagnostic test fourfold table based on Arnedos M's paper

CNB	EB		
	$+$	$-$	Total
ER$+$	251	2	253
ER$-$	4	79	83
Total	255	81	336

The result is that SEN$=98.4\%$, SPE$=97.5$, ACC$=98$, LR$+=39.36$.

(3) Relevance appraisal of diagnositc test study & the calculation and meaning of post-test probability.

Worksheet 3: Relevance appraisal of diagnostic test study

Can these results be applied to my patient care?	
Is the diagnostic test available, affordable, accurate, and precise in your setting?	
Can you generate a clinically sensible estimate of your patient's pre-test probability?	
Will the resulting post-test probabilities affect your managements and help your patients?	
Would the results of the test help your patient?	

Assumption, pretest probability (or prevalence)$=60\%$:

Pre-test odds $=$pre-test probability$/(1-$pre-test probability)
$$=0.6/(1-0.6)=1.5$$

Post-test odds$=$pre-test odds$\times$LR$=1.5\times39.36=59.04$

Post-test probability $=$post-test odds$/(1+$post-test odds)
$$=59.04/(1+59.04)=0.98$$

The post-test probability means that a patient with a positive CNB result is 98% certain to be diagnosed with the disease, in the condition of a 60% prevalence of the disease. The post-test probability can also be obtained by using LR nomogram.

Li Hongmei

第 9 章

预后性研究的严格评价

第一部分　教　学　要　求

此教学环节主要介绍预后研究的概况、影响预后的因素和生存分析。着重让学生通过临床案例分析以及互动环节掌握预后研究真实性、重要性和相关性（适用性）的评价。

1. 教学目的

掌握预后的概念，以及评价预后证据的真实性、重要性和相关性。

2. 学习目标

通过此环节的学习，学生能够：
（1）知晓预后研究的基本概念。
（2）明白什么是适合预后问题的预后研究设计类型。
（3）了解影响疾病预后的因素。
（4）认识预后指标和评价方法。
（5）严格评价预后性研究。

3. 教学方法

此环节采用讲授法、PPT 演示和互动教学法，互动教学技术包括 TPS、教师讲故事、回忆—总结—提问—联系—评论、波浪、分层蛋糕讨论和一分钟作文等。

4. 阅读材料

Henschke N，Maher C G，Refshauge K M，et al. Prognosis in patients with recent onset low back pain in Australian primary care：inception cohort study. BMJ，2008，337(7662)：154－157.

第二部分　教学设计——2 课时（80 分钟）

"预后性研究的严格评价"教学设计

序号	内　容	互动技术/教学技术	描　　　　述	时间（分钟）
1	预后简介	互动 9.1：TPS	在真实的临床实践中，经常需要考虑预后的问题。因此，对预后证据的分析和评价在临床实践中是非常重要的	10
2	讨论临床案例	互动 9.2：教师讲故事、回忆—总结—提问—联系—评论	用一个临床案例引入预后研究的评价要点	15
3	预后研究要点	PPT 演示	介绍预后研究的重点内容：样本的代表性、随访的完整性和结局指标的标准	10
4	预后研究真实性和重要性评价	互动 9.3：波浪和分层蛋糕讨论	采用 wave 技术将学生分组后，学生阅读指定的文献，小组讨论，完成小组任务：评价预后研究的真实性并完成评价工作表 1	30
5	生存分析简介	PPT 演示	介绍生存分析，包括生存率、中位生存时间和生存曲线	10
6	小结和课后作业	互动 9.4：一分钟作文和课后作业	请大家用一分钟写出教师给出问题的答案。课后请继续阅读论文，并讨论预后研究的重要性评价和相关性评价。完成评价工作表 2～3，并在下一次课前提交	5

第三部分　教　学　内　容

1. 预后简介

互动 9.1：TPS

　　教师：在真实的临床实践中，无论是患者、同事，还是我们自己，我们经常需要考虑预后的问题。例如：

（1）"我将会发生什么事？"（一个刚被诊断出患有老年痴呆症的患者可能会问）

（2）"检测出有尿微量白蛋白的患者是否会影响他的预后？"（内科医生问）

（3）"乳腺癌Ⅱ期的患者手术后的生存时间是多长？"（外科医生问）

为什么我们会对预后的问题感兴趣呢？请同学们思考，与同伴讨论，然后与全班分享。

学生1：患者和家属想知道在疾病进展过程中会发生什么、生存和生活质量如何。

学生2：患者不仅希望要活着，而且要高质量地生活。

学生3：正确评估每一个患者的预后情况可以提高医疗水平。

教师：如果你是一个临床医生，你认为哪些因素会影响预后？请各位思考，与同伴讨论并与全班分享。

学生4：患者的年龄和性别。

学生5：治疗的方法和药物。

学生6：疾病的病程和严重程度。

教师：非常好！ 大家回答的都很好。在临床实践中，预后因素多种多样，包括筛查、早期诊断、积极治疗等，可能会影响疾病的全过程。通常情况下，相同疾病和相似情况的患者会有不同的结局。因此，对预后证据的分析和评价在临床实践中是非常重要的。

（1）预后：是指预测某些特定情况的患者将来可能发生的情况，以及预测疾病不同结局的影响因素。

（2）预后研究：使用变量来分析、确定重要预测指标，并提供关于疾病结局的概率的研究（结局包括治愈/控制/复发/恶化/残障/并发症/死亡等）。

（3）预后研究的预测指标：治愈率、控制率、死亡率、生存时间等。

（4）预后研究常用的研究设计：有几种研究设计类型可以提供预后信息。例如，干预性的随机对照试验可以提供对照组和干预组某些结局指标的预后信息；观察性研究如病例对照研究和队列研究常用于观察特定疾病的预后因素；队列研究有不同的形式，可以是回顾性的，也可以是前瞻性的。

2. 临床案例讨论

互动9.2： 教师讲故事、回忆—总结—提问—联系—评论

教师：接下来，我想用一个临床案例引入我们今天的课程。

　　珍妮,35 岁,主诉腰痛。患者自述几天前在整理床铺的时候,感觉到右侧腰部(就在右侧髂骨上方)尖锐的"刺痛"。疼痛刚开始的那一天,她坚持去上班,但她后来不得不又回来了。她描述疼痛呈钝痛[疼痛数字评分量表(NRS)评分 2,2/10],偶尔也会在活动时出现尖锐的疼痛(4/10),无放射痛。她发现热敷可以暂时减轻疼痛。检查没有发现什么异常。珍妮尚未至其他的医疗机构接受治疗。她想知道如果疼痛无限地继续下去后果会有多严重。

　　请仔细阅读上述临床案例并回答问题:这个临床案例属于什么类型的问题? 治疗? 诊断试验? 危险因素/病因? 还是预后?

　　学生: 预后。

　　教师: 请回忆之前学过的内容,告诉我循证医学的五个步骤是什么?

　　学生: 提出可回答的问题;检索证据;评价证据;应用证据和评估后效。

　　教师: 答得对。评价证据是我们今天学习的重点。首先,请构建 PICO 的问题。请边写边思考:预后研究中,PICO 分别代表什么?

　　学生:(构建 PICO 问题)

P(患者/人群)	
I(干预)	
C(对照措施)	
O(结局指标)	

　　教师: 构建预后研究问题最简单的形式需要包括两个部分:患者和结局指标。

　　不同的研究问题需要不同的研究设计。回答有关预后的问题,哪种研究设计更好?

　　学生: 系统评价(SR)。

　　教师: 很显然,SR 是回答我们临床问题的最好的证据,就像我们之前学过的。但在目前,预后研究相关的 SR 很少见,在这一章我们将重点讨论单个的研究。队列研究是目前公认的回答预后问题的最佳设计方案。

　　(1)疾病预后研究常用的设计方案:疾病预后研究包括预后因素的研究及预后的评估,根据研究的目的及可行性原则,可选择的研究设计方案包括描述性研究、病例对照研究、队列研究和试验性研究，但预后研究的最佳研究方案是队列研究（包括前瞻性的和回顾性的）。随机对照研究可以用于预后研究，但往往因为研究对象有严格的纳入标准，所以对全体患者的代表性较差。病例对照研究常用于罕见疾病或需要长期随访疾病的预后研究，但因为该研究设计方案容易发生选择性偏倚和测量偏倚，所以结论的证据强度不够强。

（2）队列研究：队列研究将受试人群分为两组，一组接受暴露，另一组不接受。从暴露到结局方向进行观察，以获得感兴趣的结局。

3. 预后研究的要点

（1）样本的代表性：理想情况下，预后研究所纳入的样本应该是所有患同一疾病的患者，且都从其患病开始进行研究。但实际上，这样理想的预后研究不可能得到，因此，为了获得一个尽可能理想的证据，首先要分析研究中的对象的定义是否严格，这些对象是否能代表该类疾病的患者人群，即预后研究应该包括明确的诊断标准、纳入标准和排除标准。

（2）随访的完整性：理想的情况下，所有患者应随访至痊愈或至疾病的某个结局。如果随访时间较短，只有少部分患者出现了我们想考察的结局，我们将无法获得足够的信息来为患者提供建议。在这种情况下，我们最好寻找其他证据。相比之下，如果经过数年的随访，只有少数不良事件发生，这种研究显示的良好预后结果非常有助于让患者安心。

如何判断"随访完整"呢？目前尚无统一标准，一般我们采用两种判断方法。第一种简单的方法是"5 和 20"规则：即失访率小于 5% 时，产生的偏倚较小；大于 20% 时，则严重影响结果的真实性；失访率介于 5%～20% 之间时，研究结果比较可靠。第二种方法是可以考虑"最佳"和"最差"的情况，称为"敏感性分析"。

（3）结局评定标准的客观性：疾病在许多重要方面影响着患者，有些很容易被发现，有些则比较微妙。一般来说，两种情况的结局——死亡或完全康复——相对容易确认。介于这两个极端之间的是一系列更难以检测或确认的结局（如残疾、复发和生活质量的变化等）。研究人员必须在研究开始前提供明确的结局定义和客观的测量标准。客观标准可以避免研究人员在判断预后结局时产生分歧，从而影响预后研究的结论。但是即使有了客观的标准，如果结局是功能性的或主观性的指标，也可能会出现一些偏差。因此，"死亡"和"残疾"等结局可以不采用盲法，一些基于主观印象的预后结局则应该使用盲法，如疼痛程度的等级。通过盲法，可以严格防止测量偏倚的影响。

4. 预后研究真实性和重要性评价

互动 9.3：波浪和分层蛋糕讨论

教师：现在让我们放松一下,做一个波浪活动。请同学们从 1 到 5 依次报数,记住自己的号码。

学生：(报数)

教师：很好。现在,请号码为 1 的所有同学起立,请坐下。请号码为 2 所有起立,好,坐下。号码为 3 的请起立,请坐。号码为 4 的请起立,请坐。号码为 5 的,请坐。非常好！现在我们请每一组同学依次起立、坐下,像波浪一样,每组同学起立时同时叫出自己的号码,并高举双臂,现在开始。

学生：(做波浪)

教师：现在我们把相同号码的同学作为一个小组,每个小组找一张桌子围坐下,请阅读我分发的这篇文献,阅读完和小组成员讨论预后证据的真实性和重要性。

Henschke N,Maher C G,Refshauge K M,et al. Prognosis in patients with recent onset low back pain in Australian primary care: inception cohort study. BMJ,2008,337(7662):154-157.

学生：(阅读和讨论)

教师：(给每个小组发放一张纸、一支笔和一份粘胶,保证每组笔的颜色不同。)请大家完成评价工作表,并将其贴在黑板上。每小组推选一位代表,向全班解释你们的表格。

工作表 1：预后研究的真实性评价

预后研究的证据是否真实有效？	
1. 是否有代表性且定义明确的患者样本群体,并都在病程相同起点开始随访？	
2. 研究对象的随访时间是否足够长,随访是否完整？	
3. 对结果的评定标准是否客观,没有偏倚？	
4. 如果有亚组的不同预后： 是否对重要的预后因素进行了校正？ 是否对"测试组"的自变量(x)进行了校正？	

5. 生存分析

（1）生存率：在某一时间点的生存百分数（如 1 年生存率、5 年生存率）。

（2）中位生存时间：即观察到 50% 的研究对象死亡所需随访的时间。

（3）生存曲线：在不同时间点上，研究样本没有发生该结果（死亡）的比例（通常以百分数表示）。在预后研究中我们常绘制成的生存曲线是 Kaplan-Meier 曲线。下图显示了四种生存曲线，每一种曲线的结论都不一样。

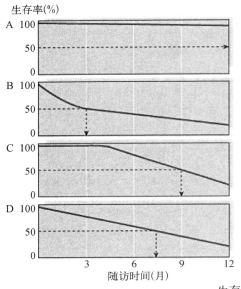

A: 从始至终没有发现死亡，说明该病预后良好；或随访时间太短，还没有发现死亡患者。
B: 该病早期预后差，3 个月后生存率缓慢下降，中位生存时间为 3 个月，1 年生存率为 20%。
C: 该病早期预后较好，5 个月后迅速恶化，中位生存时间 9 个月，1 年生存率为 20%。
D: 随着时间推移，该病生存率稳步下降，中位生存时间大概是 7.5 个月，1 年的生存率为 20%。

生存曲线

6. 小结和课后作业

互动 9.4：一分钟作文

教师： 这堂课很快就要结束了，请大家用一分钟时间写下以下问题的答案："你今天学到的最重要的东西是什么？"

学生：（思考和书写）

互动 9.5：课后作业

教师： 课后请继续阅读论文，并讨论预后证据的重要性评价。每一个小组完成评价工作表 2~3,并在下一次课的时候提交。评价表由两部分组成:"预后研究的证据是否具备重要性?"和"我们能把真实的,重要的证据应用到患者身上吗?"

工作表 2　预后研究的重要性评价

预后研究的证据是否具备重要性?	
1.在一定时间内,所研究结果发生的可能性有多大?	
2.预后估计的精确度如何?	

工作表 3　预后研究的相关性评价

我们能把真实的、重要的证据应用到患者身上吗?	
1.研究的对象和我们所遇到的病例是否相似?	
2.研究结果是否有助于对临床治疗做出决策和对患者进行解释?	

王俊瑛

Chapter 9

Critical Appraisal of Prognostic Studies

Part I Teaching Requirements

This session is an introduction to prognosis, key issues for prognosis studies and survival analysis. It emphasizes the validity, importance and relevance (applicability) of the prognosis studies through clinical scenario and interactive teaching techniques.

1. Teaching aims

Students should be able to grasp the concept of prognosis, and appraise the validity, importance and relevance of prognostic evidence.

2. Learning objectives

After completing this session, students should be able to:

(1) Know about the basic concept of prognosis study.

(2) Understand what types of study designs are appropriate for evaluating clinical questions about prognosis.

(3) Understand the influencing factors associated with studies of prognosis.

(4) Recognize the assessment indicators and methods for prognosis studies.

(5) Critically appraise prognostic studies.

3. Teaching methods

This session will use lecture, PPT presentation and interactive teaching method. Interactive teaching techniques including TPS, instructor storytelling, recall-summarize-question-connect-comment, wave, layered cake discussion, one-minute papers and others.

4. Reading materials

Henschke N, Maher C G, Refshauge K M, et al. Prognosis in patients with recent onset low back pain in Australian primary care: inception cohort study. BMJ, 2008, 337(7662): 154 - 157.

Part II　Teaching Design — 2 periods (80 minutes)

Teaching design of "Critical Appraisal of Prognostic Studies"

No.	Content	Interactive technique/teaching techniques	Descriptions	Time (minutes)
1	Introduction to prognosis	Interaction 9.1: TPS	In real clinical situation, prognosis is often a concern. Therefore, the analysis and evaluation of prognostic evidence is very important in clinical practice.	10
2	Discussion on clinical scenario	Interaction 9.2: Instructor storytelling, recall-summarize-question-connect-comment	Use a clinical scenario as an example in the following lecture. Introduce some key issues of appraising prognosis studies.	15
3	key issues for prognosis studies	PPT presentation	Introduce the key issues for prognosis studies: representative of sample, completion of follow-up and outcome criteria.	10
4	Appraise the evidence about prognosis valid and important	Interaction 9.3: Wave, layered cake discussion PPT presentation	Use wave technique to classify students into groups. Students read the assigned article, discuss the issues within the group, and then complete the group task: appraise the validity of prognosis evidence and complete the appraisal worksheet1.	30
5	Introduction to survival analysis	PPT presentation	Introduce survival analysis, including survival rate, median survival time and survival curves.	10

(continued)

No.	Content	Interactive technique/ teaching techniques	Descriptions	Time (minutes)
6	Summary and homework	Interaction 9. 4: One-minute papers and homework	Everyone writes answers to a specific question in one minute. Keep on reading the paper and appraising the importance of prognosis evidence after class and hand in the appraisal Worksheet 2 – 3 before next class.	5

Part III Teaching Contents

1. Introduction to prognosis

Interaction 9.1: TPS

Teacher: In real clinic situation, whether it is posed by our patients, colleagues or ourselves, we frequently need to consider the questions about prognosis, for example:

(1) "What's going to happen to me?" (A patient newly diagnosed with Alzheimer's dementia might ask.)

(2) "Should a patient with urine m-Alb will affect his prognosis?" (A physician asks.)

(3) "What is the survival time of a patient with stage II breast cancer after operation?" (A surgeon asks.)

Why should we be interested in prognosis? Please think about it and talk it with your parters and share it in the class.

Student 1: Patients and their family members want to know what will happen to them, in terms of disease progression, survival and the quality of life.

Student 2: The patient hopes not only to live, but also a high-quality of life.

Student 3: A correct evaluation of the prognosis on each patient can improve the level of medical treatment.

Teacher: If you were a clinician, which factors do you think will affect prognosis? Please think, discuss and then share your opinions in class.

Student 4: Patient's age and gender.

Student 5: Treatment and medicine.

Student 6: The course and severity of the disease.

Teacher: Great! Your answers are very good. In clinical practice, there are many prognostic factors that include screening, early diagnosis, active treatments and others, and that may influence the whole course of the disease. It often occurs that patients with the same disease and similar conditions have quite different outcomes. Therefore, analysis and evaluation of prognostic evidence is very important in clinical practice.

(1) Prognosis: Prognosis is to predict what is likely to happen to a patient with certain characteristics and what are the influencing factors of various outcomes of the disease.

(2) Prognostic study: Using variable approach in design and analysis to determine the important predictors of the studied outcomes and to provide outcome probabilities (cured/under control/recurrence/deterioration/disability/complication/death ...).

(3) Indicators in prognostic study: Cure rate, control rate, mortality rate, survival time, etc.

(4) Commonly-used study design in prognosis: Several different types of study design can provide prognostic information. For example, randomized controlled trials of interventions may provide prognostic information on certain outcomes in the control and intervention groups. Observational studies, like case-control studies and cohort studies, can be used to examine prognostic factors in relation to particular diseases. Cohort studies can take several forms; for example, they may be retrospective or prospective.

2. Discussion on clinical scenario

Interaction 9.2: Instructor storytelling, recall-summarize-question-connect-comment

Teacher: Next, I would like to use a clinical scenario as an example to lead our following lecture.

Jenny is 35 years old, complaining of low back pain. She related that the pain began a few days ago while she was making her bed and felt a sharp "stab" in her right lower back (just above the right iliac crest). She tried to go to work on the day the episode started, but she has since returned. She describes the pain as a dull and achy [numberal rating scale (NRS) score 2, 2/10] and occasionally sharp (4/10) pain depending on her movements but it did not radiate. She had been finding that a hot pack gave her some temporary relief. Exam findings were unremarkable. Jenny had not gone to any other provider to seek treatment yet. She wanted to know how serious this pain was, if she would continue to have it indefinitely.

Please read the clinical scenario carefully and answer the questions.

Which type of question is the clinical scenario about? Therapy? Diagnostic test? Risk factors/Etiology? Prognosis?

Student: Prognosis.

Teacher: Please recall what you learned before and tell me: what are the five steps in EBM?

Student: Ask an answerable questions; acquire the evidence; appraise the evidence; apply the evidence and assess your performance.

Teacher: That's right. Appraising the evidence is the key point of today's study. Firstly, please try to build a PICO. Please write and think about the following question: for a prognostic study, what does PICO stand for seperatelly?

Student: (build a PICO)

P (Patient/Population)	
I (Intervention)	
C (Comparison)	
O (Outcome)	

> **Teacher:** Two parts are needed to construct the simplest form of prognostic study: patient and outcome.
>
> Different research issues require different study designs. To answer the questions about prognosis, what kind of study design is better?
>
> **Student:** Systematic review (SR).
>
> **Teacher:** Obviously, SR is the best evidence which may answer our clinical questions as we learned before. But so far, relevant SR of prognosis studies are rare and we'll focus the discussion in this chapter on single studies. Cohort studies represent the best design for answering prognosis questions.

(1) Research designs of prognosis study: Disease prognosis research includes the study of prognostic factors and the assessment of prognosis. According to the purpose and feasibility principle of the study, research design options include descriptive study, case control study, cohort study and experimental study, but the best research design for prognosis is cohort study (includes prospective and retrospective studies). Randomized controlled studies can be used in prognostic studies, but they tend to be less representative of the total patient population because of the strict inclusion criteria. Case-control studies are often used to study the prognosis of rare diseases or diseases requiring long-term follow-up, but because the study design is prone to selective bias and measurement bias, the evidence for conclusions is not strong enough.

(2) Cohort study: Two groups (cohorts) of patients are identified, with one that receives the exposure of interest, and one that does not. Follow these cohorts forward for the outcome of interest occurrence.

3. Key issues for prognosis studies

(1) Representative of sample: Ideally, the prognosis study we find would include the entire population of patients who ever developed the disease, and were studied from the instant the disease developed. Unfortunately, this is impossible, and we'll have to determine how the report

we've found approximates to the ideal evidence, how the target disorder was defined and how participants were assembled. Thus, the prognosis study we find should include clear diagnostic criteria, inclusion criteria and exclusion criteria.

(2) Follow-up completes: Ideally, every patient in the cohort would be followed until they fully recover or develop one of the disease outcomes. If follow-up is too short, it may occur that a few patients develop the outcome of interest and therefore we could not get enough information to help us to provide some medical suggestion for our patients. On this occasion, we'd better look for other evidence. In contrast, if after years of follow-up, only a few adverse events have occurred, this good prognostic result is very useful in reassuring our patients about their future.

How can we judge whether follow-up is "sufficiently complete"? There is no single answer to all the studies, but we offer two approaches to help you. The first way we suggest is considering the simple "5 and 20" rule: fewer than 5% loss rate probably leads to little bias, greater than 20% loss rate seriously threatens validity, and the results are reliable when the loss rate is between 5% and 20%. Secondly, we could consider the "best" and "worst" case in an approach that we call a "sensitivity analysis".

(3) Objectivity of outcome criteria: Diseases affect patients in many important ways, some are easy to spot and some are subtler. In general, outcomes at both extremes — death or full recovery — are relatively easy to confirm. In between these extremes are a wide range of outcomes that can be more difficult to detect or confirm (e.g., disability, recurrence, and changes in quality of life). Investigators will have to provide a clear definition of outcome and objective measurement criteria before the study begins. Objective criterion is to avoid differences in the determination of these outcomes by researchers, thus affecting the conclusions of prognostic studies. But even with objective criteria, some bias might creep in if the outcome is a functional or subjective indicator. Therefore, the outcomes, such as "death" and "disability", can be determined without blinding, while determination of some prognostic outcomes based on subjective impressions should be blinding, such as the degree of pain. With blinding, the influence of measurement bias could be strictly prevented.

4. Appraise the evidence about prognosis validity and importance

Interaction 9.3 : Wave and layered cake discussion

Teacher: Let us do a wave activity. Now I need you to count out from 1 to 5 one by one. Please be sure to remember the number of yours.

Students: (count out the numbers)

Teacher: Ok, all number 1 students stand up please, sit down please. all number 2, sit down please, number 3, and 4, and 5. Great! Now I want the first number, that is all number 1, of course, stand up and raise your hands and call out your number in the meantime, and sit down before the next group stands up, number by number as one falls another rises just like waves.

Students: (do the wave)

Teacher: We have 5 groups now, the same number will be in the same group. Every group please find a table, and sit down, then read the following paper and appraise the validity and importance of prognostic evidence.

Henschke N, Maher C G, Refshauge K M, et al. Prognosis in patients with recent onset low back pain in Australian primary care: inception cohort study. BMJ, 2008, 337(7662): 154 – 157.

Students: (read and discuss)

Teacher: (Distribute papers, pens and stickers to groups, different group with different color.) I need every group to complete the appraisal worksheet 1 and paste it on the blackboard. A student chosen from each group has to explain your answer in front of the class.

Worksheet 1: Validity appraisal of prognosis study

Is this evidence about prognosis valid?	
1. Was a defined, representative sample of patients assembled at a common point in the course of their disease?	
2. Was the follow-up of the study patients sufficiently long and complete?	
3. Were objective outcome criteria applied in a blind fashion?	
4. If subgroups with different prognosis are identified: was there adjustment for important prognostic factors? was there a validation in an independent "test set" patients (x)?	

5. Survival analysis

(1) Survival rate: refers to the percentage of survial at a particular point in time (such as 1-year or 5-year survival rates).

(2) Median survival time: the length of follow-up by which 50% of study patients have died.

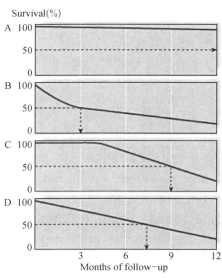

A: No patients have had events by the end of the study, which could mean that either prognosis is very good for this target disorder or the study is too short.
B: Poor prognosis early, then slower increase in mortality, with median survival time of 3 months, the proportion of patients surviving to 1 year (20%).
C: Good prognosis early, then worsening after 5 months, with median survival time of 9 months, proportion of patients surviving to 1 year (20%).
D: Steady prognosis, with median survival time of approximately 7.5 months, proportion of patients surviving to 1 year (20%).

Survival curve

(3) Survival curves: survival curves depict, at each point in time, the proportion (expressed as a percentage) of the original study sample who have not yet had a specified outcome (death). In prognosis studies we often find results presented as Kaplan-Meier curve, which is a type of survival curve. The following figure shows four survival curves, each leading to a different conclusion.

6. Summary and homework

Interaction 9.4: One-minute paper

Teacher: The class will be over soon, everyone writes for one minute on a specific question "what is the most important thing you learned today?"

Students: (think and write)

Interaction 9.5 : Homework

Teacher: Keep on reading the paper and appraising the importance of prognosis evidence after class. I need every group to complete and hand in the appraisal Worksheet 2 - 3 before the next class. The worksheet consists of two parts: "Is this valid evidence about prognosis important?" and "Can we apply this valid, important evidence about prognosis to our patient?"

worksheet 2: Importance appraisal of prognosis study

Is this valid evidence about prognosis important?	
1. How likely are the outcomes to happen over time?	
2. How precise are the prognostic estimates?	

worksheet 3: Relevance appraisal of prognosis study

Can we apply this valid, important evidence about prognosis to our patient?	
1. Is our patient so different from those in the study?	
2. Will this evidence make a clinically important impact on our conclusions about what to offer or to tell our patients?	

Wang Junying

第 10 章

系统评价与 Meta 分析

第一部分 教 学 要 求

本次课程第一部分是关于一个模拟的案例,这个案例可以考虑使用系统评价/Meta 分析。第二部分是让学生通过角色扮演来强化什么情况下可以使用系统评价/Meta 分析。第三部分是通过小讲座回答第一部分提出的问题并分享系统评价/Meta 分析的要点。第四部分是通过一个短小的讲座,介绍如何设计系统评价/Meta 分析。第五部分是通过一个真实的案例,分享系统评价/Meta 分析论文摘要中的要点。

1. 教学目的

分享系统评价/Meta 分析的定义、基本要素,包括系统评价/Meta 分析的目的、方法、结果和结论。

2. 学习目标

通过此环节的学习,学生能够:

(1) 给系统评价/Meta 分析下定义。

(2) 描述何时需要实施或者检索系统评价/Meta 分析。

(3) 列出系统评价/Meta 分析的优势。

(4) 列出系统评价/Meta 分析的不足。

3. 教学方法

此环节采用讲授法、PPT 演示和互动教学法,互动教学技术包括模拟案例、角色扮演、个案教学和问卷调查。

4. 阅读材料

(1) Kydd A S,Seth R,Buchbinder R,et al. Uricosuric medications for

chronic gout. Cochrane Database Syst Rev，2014，（11）：CD010457. doi：10.1002/14651858.CD010457.pub2.PubMed PMID：25392987.

（2）Seth R，Kydd A S，Buchbinder R，et al. Allopurinol for chronic gout. Cochrane Database Syst Rev，2014，（10）：CD006077. doi：10.1002/14651858.CD006077.pub3.Review.PubMed PMID：25314636.

（3）Higgins J P T，Thomas J，Chandler J，et al. Cochrane handbook for systematic reviews of interventions version 6.0（updated July 2019）. Cochrane，2019. http：//www.training.cochrane.org/handbook［2020 - 02 - 02］.

（4）Moher D，Liberati A，Tetzlaff J，et al. Preferred reporting items for systematic reviews and Meta-analyses：the PRISMA statement. PLoS Med 6（7）：e1000097. http：//journals.plos.org/plosmedicine/article?id＝10.1371/journal.pmed.1000097［2020 - 02 - 02］.

第二部分　教学设计——2 课时（80 分钟）

"系统评价与 Meta 分析"教学设计表

序号	内　容	互动技术/ 教学技术	描　　　述	时间 （分钟）
1	热身	互动 12.1：分享模拟案例并提问	分享一个模拟案例：几个研究关注同样的疾病(高尿酸血症)和干预方法,但是结果不同 提问：作为医生,我们遇到这样的问题该怎么办？	10
2	什么时候需要考虑用系统评价/Meta 分析?	互动 12.2：角色扮演	1. 招募 3 名志愿者,分别扮演医生和患者,来回答上述问题 2. 请志愿者用 3 分钟来准备表演,其余的学生思考如何回答上述问题 3. 请志愿者表演 4. 教师请观众反馈他们看到了什么、听到了什么、有什么感想	20
3	介绍系统评价/Meta 分析	PPT 演示	1. 分享在现实中医生如何基于系统评价/Meta 分析的结果解答上述案例中的问题 2. 为学生提供系统评价/Meta 分析的关键知识点	10
4	如何设计系统评价/Meta 分析?	PPT 演示	为学生们提供如何设计系统评价/Meta 分析的信息	10

（续表）

序号	内　容	互动技术/ 教学技术	描　　述	时间 （分钟）
5	如何实施系统评价/Meta 分析？	互动 12.3：个案教学	1. 招募 4 个小组的志愿者，每个小组 4 人 2. 给各小组分配任务，分别报告一篇期刊论文的目的、方法、结果和结论。每个小组有 7 分钟的时间准备，2 分钟汇报 3. 请其他学生思考上述论文的目的、方法、结果和结论 4. 四个小组分别汇报他们的发现。教师请班上学生说说他们有什么想法	25
6	课后调查	互动 12.4：问卷调查	分发和回收课后调查问卷，调查学生们对该门课程的掌握程度和态度（问卷见附录Ⅰ）	5

第三部分　教 学 内 容

1. 热身

模拟案例：如何回答下列问题？

假如我们有一个研究，关于用两个药物（M1 和 M2）降低高尿酸血症患者的血尿酸水平。这个研究是随机对照试验设计的，结果显示 M1 效果比 M2 好。但是其他 6 个一样的研究，有的显示 M1 比 M2 好，有的显示 M2 比 M1 好。作为医生我们应该怎么办呢？

互动 10.1：分享案例并提问

教师：我们说，循证医学是基于证据来帮助患者，而证据从哪里来呢？（说完，稍停，用身体语言表示期待学生回应，看看学生有没有反馈。）

学生 1：证据从……中来。（只要学生没有提到证据的来源之一是科学研究，我们可以按照下面第二种情况来继续往下走。）

学生 2：证据除了从"经验"中来以外，通常证据的常见来源是"科学研究"。（当学生给出这样的答案时，鼓励学生，认同这样的说法。）

教师：假如有个研究是这样的，有 200 个高尿酸血症患者，现在有两种药物——M1 和 M2，我们的目标是了解到底哪种药物更好？具体做法是把

200 个患者随机分成两组——M1 组,100 人,使用药物 M1,每天 1 片,30 天为 1 个疗程;M2 组 100 人,使用药物 M2,每天 1 片,30 天为 1 个疗程。在给药前对每一个患者进行抽血检测空腹血尿酸,一个疗程后的第一天对每一个患者进行抽血检测空腹血尿酸。以血尿酸值$>417\ \mu mol/L$ 为高尿酸血症,$\leq$ $417\ \mu mol/L$ 为正常。结果显示,给药前所有 200 个患者都是高尿酸血症患者;一个疗程结束后,M1 组有 100%(100/100)的患者空腹血尿酸回到正常范围,M2 组有 60%(60/100)的患者空腹血尿酸回到正常范围。经统计学检验,两组有效率有统计学差异($P<0.05$)。结论认为,药物 M1 控制血尿酸的效果优于药物 M2。

教师:请问,如果你是医生,要回答患者哪种药物更好,该怎么回答呢?

学生:×××药物更好。(如果有学生回答,鼓励! 如果没有学生回答,教师接着说,比如"很简单,是不是啊? 哪个药物的有效率更高,哪个就更好。")

教师:假设还有人在不同地方、不同时间做了跟上述试验一模一样的研究,结果如下表。粗略估计,M1 组有效率还是比 M2 组的有效率高(89%对 81%),但试验 2 和试验 4 显示相反的结果。如果研究的结果不一致,甚至得出截然相反的结论,这时候,你还能回答哪一种更好吗?(如果有人给出正确的答案,说"谢谢"。如果有人给出不正确的答案,感谢他/她的回答。教师暂时不给出答案。在角色扮演之后给出答案。)

表1　关于高尿酸血症治疗的随机对照试验的 Meta 分析

研 究	M1 组有效人数	M1 组总人数	M1 组有效率	M2 组有效人数	M2 组总人数	M2 组有效率
试验 1	100	100	100%	60	100	60%
试验 2	180	200	90%	190	200	95%
试验 3	350	380	92%	340	380	89%
试验 4	50	70	71%	60	70	86%
试验 5	890	1 000	89%	810	1 000	81%
试验 6	90	100	90%	75	100	75%
试验 7	80	100	80%	50	100	50%
共 计	1 740	1 950	89%	1 585	1 950	81%

(以分享案例的形式进行热身,会让教、学双方感到比较轻松而且效果不错。)

2. 什么时候需要考虑用系统评价/Meta 分析

互动 10.2:角色扮演

教师:我们需要 3 个志愿者(结合 PPT 上的内容,介绍志愿者需要做什么,详见教材中的表格)。愿意表演的同学请举手?(如果有足够的志愿者,很好! 感谢3个志愿者。如果没有,或者人数不足,谢谢已经报名的学生。与此同时,向全班解释一个物色志愿者的办法:你随口说一个含两位数的数字,请学号最后两位数与这个数一样的学生当志愿者,有多少个缺口,说多少个数。使用学生名册作参考。)

〔教师与3名志愿者讨论如何表演:一人当医生1,一人当医生2,一人当患者。看看如何回答刚才的问题?(教师主要关注三位志愿者的表演准备工作,如果需要教师协助,教师一定要有一些思路和指导,哪怕不是十全十美。其余的学生也要有事情做:比如左侧的任务:用眼睛看,用耳朵听,用头脑想"三位志愿者即将给出的表演"。或者,提一些问题给他们思考,比如,如果由他们来表演,他们会怎么做呢?)〕

学生:〔志愿者表演医生和患者的互动(教师作为主持人,需要提供表演"开始""时间""结束"等信息)。〕

教师:〔请一名学生来当助教,任务是用粉笔在黑板上记下观众学生说的话。教师问观众学生们看到了什么、听到了什么、有什么感想(教师指导助教在黑板上简单列出3个栏目"1. 看到的,2. 听到的,3. 感想"。教师也要问表演的学生有什么补充)。〕

感谢表演的同学、助教和观众!

是否真的是药物 M1 比药物 M2 更有效,需要用专门的 Meta 分析软件(如 RevMan 5.3)来处理。经过 RevMan 5.3 分析,结果确认 M1 组有效率比 M2 组的有效率高,详见下图所示。

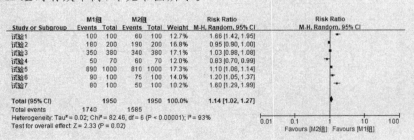

关于高尿酸血症治疗的随机对照试验的 Meta 分析(森林图)

(以角色扮演的形式目的是加深学生的印象。)

3. 介绍系统评价/Meta 分析

(1)什么是 Meta 分析:一方面 Meta 分析是一个统计学方法,汇总不同研究的结果；另一方面，Meta 分析是一种研究设计，回顾统计学上类似的研究，汇总和分析若干研究的结果。

（2）Meta 分析的优势和不足

A. 优势：① 获得更强的统计效能；② 确证性的数据分析；③ 更强的外推到总体的能力；④ 考虑基于证据的资源。

B. 不足：① 不易识别适合的研究；② 不是所有的研究都能提供完整的数据以便纳入研究和分析；③ 需要复杂的统计学技术；④ 研究人群的异质性。

（3）什么是系统评价：系统评价是一种文献综述，针对事先形成的研究问题，系统地收集、评价、选择和合成若干高质量的研究证据，借以回答相关的研究问题。

（4）系统评价的优势与不足

A. 优势：① 系统回顾现有文献和其他资源（包括未出版的文献、正在进行的研究）；② 对之前的研究进行综述相对于进行一个新的研究而言成本更小；③ 耗时较少；④ 比单个的研究有更强的推论总体的能力；⑤ 比单个的研究结果更加可靠和精确；⑥ 考虑基于证据的资源。

B. 不足：① 未出版的文献可能不容易找到；② 有时候不容易汇总数据。

4. 如何设计系统评价/Meta 分析

（1）Meta 分析的主要步骤

A. 形成研究问题。

B. 检索相关文献。

C. 选择目标文献。

D. 收集相关信息。

E. 汇总效应值。

F. 敏感性分析。

G. 估计发表偏倚。

（2）系统评价的主要步骤

A. 形成研究问题和研究方法。

B. 从符合特定标准的研究中搜索相关研究，例如，只选择质量好的研究并回答问题。

C. 提取相关数据，包括研究是如何进行的（通常称为方法或干预），谁参与了研究（包括多少人），如何支付（如资金来源）以及发生了什么（结果）。

D. 根据第一阶段研究的标准来判断数据的质量。

E. 分析和汇总数据（使用复杂的统计方法），得出所有数据的总体结果。这种数据汇总可以通过水滴图（也称森林图）来可视化。森林图中的钻石图形表示包含所有数据的汇总结果。因为这个汇总结果使用了来自多个研究的数据，而不仅仅是一个研究的数据，所以它被认为是更可靠和更好的证据。汇总的数据越多，我们对结论就越有信心。

这一步一旦完成，该综述就可能发表和传播，当其被作为证据时，就能被应用于实践。

5. 如何实施系统评价/Meta 分析

互动 10.3： 个案教学法

　　教师：我们需要做个小游戏，需要几个志愿者。哪些同学要当志愿者？要当志愿者的同学请举手。（如果有足够的志愿者，很好！感谢志愿者。分组，3～4 人/组。如果没有，或者人数不足，谢谢已经报名的学生。与此同时，向全班解释一个物色志愿者的办法：你随口说一个含两位数的数字，请学号最后两位数与这个数一样的学生当志愿者，有多少个缺口，说多少个数。使用学生名册作为参考。）

　　［教师安排 4 个志愿者小组任务，分别找出摘要里面的"目的""方法""结果"和"结论"是什么。安排全班没有当志愿者的学生一个任务：看看摘要里面的"目的""方法""结果"和"结论"分别是什么（教师主要关注 4 个志愿者小组的准备工作，如果需要教师协助，教师一定要协助。给出准备的时间，提醒还剩下的准备时间）。］

　　学生：［志愿者汇报各自的结果（教师作为主持人，需要提供汇报"开始""时间""结束"等信息，也要问观众有什么补充或者评论）。］

　　教师：（简单总结学生们做得好的地方，有待改进的地方。）

　　感谢表演的同学、助教和观众！

　　（个案教学法有两个要素：案例和对案例的讨论。一个用于个案教学的案例内容应丰富，学生在其中可以学到如何做事儿。本次互动目的是通过这个个案分析的教学活动，给学生们分析一篇论文的摘要的经历，为阅读文献做铺垫。教师需要课前准备一篇 Meta 分析的论文摘要。）

6. 课后调查/问卷调查

发放课后调查表。该表是一套专门为这门课设计的态度和知识问卷，这套包含 21 个问题的问卷见附录Ⅰ。

韦　焘

Chapter 10

Systematic Review and Meta-analysis

Part I Teaching Requirements

The first part of this session is a simulation example where a systematic review/Meta-analysis can be considered. The second part of the session is to impress the class of when to think about a systematic review/Meta-analysis through a role-play by the students. The third part of the session is to answer the question in the first part and share key information about systematic review/Meta-analysis by giving a brief presentation. The fourth part of the session is to give a short lecture about how to design a systematic review/Meta-analysis. The fifth part of the session is to share a real case with the class about key information in the abstract of a systematic review/Meta-analysis.

1. Teaching aims

To share the definition of a systematic review and Meta-analysis; the basic elements of a systematic review/Meta-analysis including its objectives, methods, results, and conclusions.

2. Learning objectives

After completing this session, students should be able to:

(1) define a systematic review and Meta-analysis.

(2) describe when to conduct or search for a systematic review and Meta-analysis.

(3) list the major advantages of a systematic review and Meta-analysis.

(4) list the limitations of a systematic review and Meta-analysis.

3. Teaching methods

This session will use lecture，PPT presentation and interactive teaching method. Interactive teaching techniques include simulation example，role play，case method and survey.

4. Reading materials

（1）Kydd A S，Seth R，Buchbinder R，et al. Uricosuric medications for chronic gout. Cochrane Database Syst Rev，2014，（11）：CD010457. doi：10.1002/14651858.CD010457.pub2. PubMed PMID：25392987.

（2）Seth R，Kydd A S，Buchbinder R，et al. Allopurinol for chronic gout. Cochrane Database Syst Rev，2014，（10）：CD006077. doi：10.1002/14651858.CD006077.pub3. Review. PubMed PMID：25314636.

（3）Higgins J P T，Thomas J，Chandler J，et al. Cochrane handbook for systematic reviews of interventions version 6.0（updated July 2019）. Cochrane，2019. http：//www.training.cochrane.org/handbook［2020－02－02］.

（4）Moher D，Liberati A，Tetzlaff J，et al. Preferred reporting items for systematic reviews and Meta-analyses：the PRISMA statement. PLoS Med 6（7）：e1000097. http：//journals.plos.org/plosmedicine/article?id＝10.1371/journal.pmed.1000097［2020－02－02］.

Part II　Teaching Design — 2 periods（80 minutes）

Teaching design of "Systematic Review/Meta-analysis"

No.	Content	Interactive technique/ teaching techniques	Descriptions	Time （minutes）
1	Warm-up	Interaction 12.1：Simulation example sharing and question	Share a simulation example about several studies focusing on the same health condition（hyperuricemia）and intervention options（M1 vs. M2）with different results. Ask a question：what should we do in this case if we are doctors?	10
2	When to consider a systematic review/Meta-analysis?	Interaction 12.2：Role play	1. Ask 3 volunteers to play a doctor and a patient respectively and answer the question above.	20

（continued）

No.	Content	Interactive technique/ teaching techniques	Descriptions	Time (minutes)
			2. Ask the volunteers to get ready for the play (3 minutes), while the rest of the students think about how to answer the question mentioned above. 3. Ask the volunteers to give their performance for the class. 4. The teacher asks the audience what they saw, what they heard of, what they think.	20
3	Introduction to systematic review/ Meta-analysis	PPT presentation	1. Show what a real doctor may do for the example above — answer it based on the result of a systematic review/Meta-analysis. 2. Provide students with key information about systematic review/Meta-analysis.	10
4	How to design a systematic review/ Meta-analysis?	PPT presentation	Provide the class with how to design a systematic review/ Meta-analysis.	10
5	How to conduct a systematic review/Meta-analysis?	Interaction 12.3: Case method	1. Have 4 groups of volunteers with 4 students in each group. 2. Assign the groups to report the objectives, methods, results, and conclusions of a journal paper to be given to the class. They have 7 minutes to get ready, and 2 minutes to report their findings. 3. Ask the rest of the students to think about the objectives, methods, results, and conclusions of the paper mentioned above. 4. Four groups report their findings. The teacher asks the whole class to comment if they like to.	25

（**continued**）

No.	Content	Interactive technique/ teaching techniques	Descriptions	Time (minutes)
6	Survey after class	Interaction 12.4: Survey	Distribute and collect the "questionnaire after class" to investigate students' mastery and attitude towards this course (questionnaire can be seen in Appendix I).	5

Part III　Teaching Contents

1. Warm-up

Simulation example: How to answer the following questions?

Suppose we have a study on the use of two drugs (M1 and M2) to lower serum uric acid levels in patients with hyperuricemia. The study design was a randomized controlled trial. The results showed that M1 had better effect than M2. But we also have other 6 studies. Some of them show that M1 is better than M2, and some others show that M2 is better than M1. What should we do as a doctor?

Interaction 10.1: Simulation example sharing and question

Teacher: Everybody knows that EBM is based on evidence to help patients, and where does the evidence come from? (After saying that, stop for a while and use body language to expect students to respond. Wait and see if students have any feedback.)

Student 1: Evidence is from … (As long as they do not mention "scientific research", just go ahead and follow the next step below.)

Student 2: In addition to the things like "experience", evidence is usually from "scientific research". (When a student gives such an answer, we need to encourage them and agree with that.)

Teacher: If there is a study like this, suppose there were 200 hyperuricemia patients, and there were two kinds of drugs — M1 and M2. Our goal was to know which drug is better. Our specific practice was to divide the 200 patients into two groups randomly — group M1, 100 people, using M1, one tablet a day, 30 days as a course of treatment; group M2 with the other 100 people, using therapy M2, one tablet a day, 30 days as a course of treatment. Before the treatment and on the first day after treatment each one takes fasting blood uric acid test. The blood uric acid levels over 417 μmol/L was set as hyperuricemia, less than or equal to 417 μmol/L as normal. The results showed that all 200 patients had hyperuricemia before the treatment; at the end of the course of treatment, 100% (100/100) of the group M1 returned to the normal range of fasting uric acid, and 60% (60/100) of the group M2 returned to the normal range of the fasting blood uric acid. Statistically, there was a significant difference between the two groups ($P<0.05$). The conclusion is that the uric acid control of M1 is better than that of M2.

Teacher: If you are a doctor, what kind of medicine do you think is better? What is your answer?

Student 1: Drug ×××× is better. (As long as there a student answers, encourage him. If no student answers, the teacher goes on, by saying, for example, "very simple, isn't it? The drug which is more efficient than the other is better.")

Teacher: If Some people did the same research as the one described above in different places and time periods, results are as following figures. It was a rough estimate that the effective rate of the group M1 was higher than that of the group M2 (89% vs. 81%), but the trial 2 and the trial 4 showed the opposite results.

Meta-analysis of randomized controlled trials on treatment of hyperuricemia

Study	Group M1			Group M2		
	No. of patients with SUA under control	No. of patients in total	Control rate	No. of patients with SUA under control	No. of patients in total	Control rate
Study 1	100	100	100%	60	100	60%
Study 2	180	200	90%	190	200	95%

(continued)

Study	Group M1			Group M2		
	No. of patients with SUA under control	No. of patients in total	Control rate	No. of patients with SUA under control	No. of patients in total	Control rate
Study 3	350	380	92%	340	380	89%
Study 4	50	70	71%	60	70	86%
Study 5	890	1 000	89%	810	1 000	81%
Study 6	90	100	90%	75	100	75%
Study 7	80	100	80%	50	100	50%
Total	1 740	1 950	89%	1 585	1 950	81%

If studies get inconsistent results, or even contradictory, which of the two drugs is better? (If someone gives the right answer, say "thank you". If someone gives an incorrect answer, thank him/her for the answer. The teacher does not give the answer right then but after the role play.)

(It is useful to warm up by sharing examples, which allows both the teacher and students to be relaxed while learning something.)

2. When to consider a systematic review/Meta-analysis?

Interaction 10.2 : Role-play

Teacher: We need three volunteers (see the table in the textbook for details on what the volunteers need to do, with the information in the PPT slides). Please raise your hands if you are willing to perform a role-play. (If there are enough volunteers. Very good! Say "thank you" to the 3 volunteers. If not, or insufficient, say "thank you" to the volunteers. At the same time, explain to the class a way to recruit volunteers: you casually say a double-digit number, anyone whose last two-digit number in their student ID is the same as the number will be asked to volunteer. The next volunteer can be recruited in the same way. Confirm the number in the student's roster.)

[Teacher discusses with the three volunteers how to do role-play: one acts as doctor A, one as doctor B, and one as a patient. Think about how to answer the question given just now. (The teacher needs to pay attention to the preparation of the three volunteers for their performance. If the teacher is required to help, he/she has to share some ideas and guidance, although our ideas are not always perfect. The rest of the students also have something to do, such as the task on the left side: to see, to listen, and to think about the performance by the three volunteers. Or, ask them some questions: for example, what would they do if they were giving the performance?)]

Student: [Volunteers do role-play, the interaction between doctors and patients. (As a master of ceremonies, the teacher needs to provide with some information about the performance, such as "begin" "time" "stop", etc.)]

Teacher: [Ask a student as an assistant, who is to record the audience's words on the blackboard with chalk. The teacher asks the audience, what they see, what they hear and what they think. (On the blackboard, the assistant simply lists 3 columns: 1. to see, 2. to hear, 3. thoughts with the tutor of the teacher's. The teacher should also ask the volunteers to add anything.)]

Thank you, all the students, assistants and spectators!

Whether M1 is more effective than M2 needs to be processed by a special Meta-analysis software (such as RevMan 5.3). After the analysis in RevMan 5.3, the result showed that the effective rate of group M1 was higher than that of group M2. See the figure below.

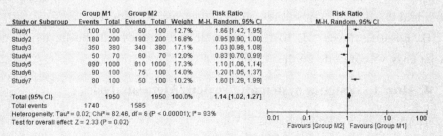

Meta-analysis of randomized controlled trials
on treatment of hyperuricemia (Forest plot)

(Role-play is to impress the students.)

3. Introduction to systematic review/Meta-analysis

（1）What is a meta analysis： On one hand，a Meta-analysis is a statistical analysis that combines the results of multiple scientific studies. On the other hand，a Meta-analysis is a survey in which the results of the studies included in the review are statistically similar and are combined and analyzed as if they were one study.

（2）Advantages and disadvantages of Meta-analysis

A. Advantages： ① greater statistical power； ② confirmatory data analysis； ③ greater ability to extrapolate to the whole； ④ consideres an evidence-based resource.

B. Disadvantages： ① difficult to identify appropriate studies； ② not all studies provide adequate data for inclusion and analysis； ③ requires advanced statistical techniques； ④ heterogeneity of study populations.

（3）What is a systematic review： A systematic review is a literature review. Focused on a single question that tries to identify，appraise，select and synthesize all high quality research evidence relevant to that question. They are designed to provide a complete，exhaustive summary of current literature relevant to a research question.

（4）Advantages and disadvantages of systematic review：

A. Advantages： ① exhaustive review of the current literature and other sources (unpublished studies，ongoing research)； ② less costly to review prior studies than to create a new study； ③ less time required than conducting a new study； ④ results can be generalized and extrapolated into the whole more broadly than individual studies； ⑤ more reliable and accurate than individual studies； ⑥ consideres an evidence-based resource.

B. Disadvantages： ① to find unpublished studies can be hard； ② may not be easy to combine studies.

4. How to design a systematic review/Meta-analysis?

（1）Steps in a Meta-analysis

A. Formulation of the research question.

B. Search of literature.

C. Selection of studies.

D. Data collection.

E. Pool the values of key variables.

F. Sensitivity analysis.

G. Estimate publication bias.

(2) Main stages of a systematic review

A. Defining a question and agreeing on an objective method.

B. A search for relevant datas from researches that match certain criteria, for example, only selecting research that is good quality and answers the defined question.

C. Extraction of relevant data. This can include how the research was done (often called the method or intervention), who participated in the research (including how many people), how it was paid for (for example, funding sources) and what happened (the outcomes).

D. Assess the quality of the data, using the criteria identified at the first stage.

E. Analyze and combine the data (using complex statistical methods) which give an overall result from all of the data. This combination of data can be visualized using a blobbogram (also called a forest plot). The diamond in the blobbogram represents the combined results of all the data included. Because this pool data comes from many sources instead of one, it's considered to be a more reliable and better evidence, as the more the data is, the more confidence the conclusions will promise.

Once these stages are complete, the review may be published, disseminated and translated into practice after being adopted as evidence.

5. How to conduct a systematic review/Meta-analysis?

Interaction 10.3 : Case method

Teacher: We need to play a small game. We need several volunteers. Who wants to be volunteers? Raise your hand if you want. (If there are enough volunteers. "Very good!" Give thanks to the volunteers. Then, start grouping, 3 - 4 persons/group. If not, or the number is insufficient, thank them for participating. At the same time, explain to the class a way to find the volunteers: you casually say a double-digit number, if the last two-digit number of the students is the same number as what you said, he/she will be the volunteers. You will say as many numbers as the vacancies. The student's roster is for reference.)

[Four volunteer groups are assigned to find out what the "purpose" "method" "result" and "conclusion" are in the abstract. Assign the whole class for a task: look at the "purpose" "method" "result" and "conclusion" in the abstract. (Teachers are mainly concerned with the preparation of the four volunteer groups. If teachers are needed, they must help. Give them time to prepare, and keep telling them the remaining time.)]

Student: [Volunteers report their results. (As a host, teachers need to provide information such as "start" "time" "end" and others. Ask the audience what supplements or comments they have.)]

Teacher: (Summarize briefly the points in which the students have done well and also the points needed to be improved.)

Thank you, all the students, assistants and spectators.

(There are two elements in case teaching method: case study and case discussion. An example of case teaching should be rich in content, and students can learn what to do in it. The purpose of this interaction is to help students acquire the experience of analyzing a paper abstract and pave the way for reading literatures through this case study. Teachers need to prepare an abstract of Meta-analysis before class.)

6. Survey/questionnaire after class

Distribute questionnaire after class. It is a set of attitude and knowledge questionnaire specially designed for this course. The 21-question questionnaire is shown in Appendix I.

Wei Tao

主要参考文献

Reference

韩久建.课堂互动活动有效性研究.安庆师范学院学报(社会科学版),2006,25(4): 112-114.

Alonso-Coello P, Montori V M, Díaz M G, et al. Values and preferences for oral antithrombotic therapy in patients with atrial fibrillation: physician and patient perspectives. Health Expect. 2015, 18(6): 2318-2327.

Arnedos M, Nerurkar A, Osin P, et al. Discordance between core needle biopsy (CNB) and excisional biopsy (EB) for estrogen receptor (ER), progesterone receptor (PgR) and HER2 status in early breast cancer (EBC). Annals of Oncology Official Journal of the European Society for Medical Oncology, 2009, 20(12): 1948.

Arthur B, VanGundy Pfeiffer. 101 activities for teaching creativity and problem solving. European Journal of Operational Research, 2006, 172(3): 1067-1068.

Beausoleil M. Effect of a fermented milk combining *Lactobacillus acidophilus* Cl1285 and *Lactobacillus casei* in the prevention of antibiotic-associated diarrhea: a randomized, double-blind, placebo-controlled trial. Can J Gastroenterol, 2007, 21(11): 732-736.

Covell D G, Uman G C, Manning P R. Information needs in office practice: are they being met? Ann Intern Med, 1985, 103: 596-599.

Dicenso A, Bayley L, Haynes R B. Accessing pre-appraised evidence: fine tuning 5S model into the 6S model. Evidence Based Nursing, 2009, 151(6): 99-101.

Guyatt G H, Sackett D L, Cook D J, et al. Users' guides to the medical literature: II. How to use an article about therapy or prevention: A. Are the results of the study valid? Jama, 1993, 270(21): 2598-2601.

Guyatt G, Rennie D. User's guide to the medical literature: essentials of evidence-based clinical practice. Chicago: AMA Pewaa, 2001: 3-22.

Haynes R B. Of studies, summaries, synopses, and systems: the "4S" evolution of services for finding current best evidence. Acp Journal Club, 2001, 134(2): A11.

Haynes R B. Of studies, syntheses, synopses, summaries, and systems: the "5S" evolution of information services for evidence-based health care decisions. Acp Journal Club, 2005, 145(3): A8.

Henschke N, Maher C G, Refshauge K M, et al. Prognosis in patients with recent onset low back pain in Australian primary care: inception cohort study. BMJ, 2008, 337(7662):

154－157.

Higgins J P T，Thomas J，Chandler J，et al. Cochrane handbook for systematic reviews of interventions version 6.0（updated July 2019）. Cochrane，2019. http://www.training. cochrane.org/handbook［2020－02－02］.

Kydd A S，Seth R，Buchbinder R，et al. Uricosuric medications for chronic gout. Cochrane Database Syst Rev，2014，（11）：CD010457. doi：10.1002/14651858.CD010457. pub2. PubMed PMID：25392987.

Lily A. Arya，Deborah L. Myers，et al. Dietary caffeine intake and the risk for detrusor instability：a case-control study. Obstetrics & Guynecology，2000，96（1）：85－89.

Maclean S，Mulla S，Akl E A，et al. Patient values and preferences in decision making for antithrombotic therapy：a systematic review：antithrombotic therapy and prevention of thrombosis，9th ed：American college of chest physicians evidence-based clinical practice guidelines. Chest，2012，141（2）：e1S－23S.

Morrison-Shetlar A，Marwitz M. Teaching creatively：ideas in action. Eden Prairie：Outernet，2001.

Moher D，Liberati A，Tetzlaff J，et al. Preferred reporting items for systematic reviews and Meta-analyses：The PRISMA statement. PLoS Med，6（7）：e1000097. http://journals. plos.org/plosmedicine/article?id＝10.1371/journal.pmed.1000097［2020－02－02］.

Murad M H，Asi N，Alsawas M，et al. New evidence pyramid. Evidence-based Medicine，2016，21（4）：125－127.

Richardson W S，Wilson M C，Nishikawa J，et al. The well-built clinical question：a key to evidence-based decisions. Acp Journal Club，1995，123（3）：A12.

Sackett D L，et al. Evidence based medicine：what it is and what it isn't. BMJ，1996，3（12）：12.

Seth R，Kydd A S，Buchbinder R，et al. Allopurinol for chronic gout. Cochrane Database Syst Rev，2014，（10）：CD006077. doi：10.1002/14651858.CD006077. pub3. Review. PubMed PMID：25314636.

Silberman M. Active Learning：101 strategies to teach any subject. Adult Education，1996：189.

Straus S E，Richardson W S，Glasziu P，et al. Evidence-based medicine：how to practice and teach EMB. 3th ed. Singapore：Elsevier（Singapore）Pte Ltd.，2006.

Thomas A，Angelo K. Classroom assessment techniques. 2nd Edition. San Francisco：Jossey-Bass，1993.

Volk R J，Llewellyn-Thomas H，Stacey D，et al. Ten years of the International Patient Decision Aid Standards Collaboration：evolution of the core dimensions for assessing the quality of patient decision aids. Bmc Medical Informatics & Decision Making，2013，13 Suppl 2（S2）：S1.

Watkins，Ryan. 75 E-learning activities：making online learning interactive. Personnel Psychology，2005，59（1）：269－271.

附录 I

问　　卷

课　前　问　卷

专业　　　　　　　班级　　　　　　　性别

同学们,大家好!此问卷是为了解同学们的学习状况和需求,不会影响考试成绩,请如实填写。每一问题后均有若干选项,请在符合自己情况的选项前打勾,相容性的选项可多选。

一、对课程的了解

1. 学习本课程前是否对其进行了解和预习?
   A. 有　　　　　　　　　B. 没有

2. 听到课程名称,你对这门课感兴趣吗?
   A. 非常感兴趣　　　　　　　　B. 还是想了解一些
   C. 无所谓　　　　　　　　　　D. 不感兴趣

3. 你对"循证医学"了解多少?
   A. 较多　　　　　　　　　　　B. 了解一些
   C. 听说过　　　　　　　　　　D. 没听说过,不了解

4. 说到"循证医学",你联想到的是?
   A. 查文献　　　　　　　　　　B. Meta 分析和随机对照试验
   C. 依据证据的临床决策　　　　D. 没什么联想

5. 你觉得循证医学会对你将来的工作和学习有用吗?
   A. 非常有用　　B. 应该有用　　C. 没有什么用　　D. 不知道

6. 流行病学是研究?
   A. 传染病的诊断和治疗
   B. 流行病的诊断和治疗
   C. 特定人群中疾病、健康状况的分布及其决定因素
   D. 不知道

7. 对统计学知识的了解程度是?
    A. 较多
    B. 了解一些
    C. 听说过
    D. 没听说过,不了解
8. 对文献检索知识和技能的了解程度是?
    A. 学得很好,能检索到想要的信息
    B. 一般
    C. 考试过了就忘记了
    D. 没听说过,不了解
9. 你参加过或正在参加科研课题吗?
    A. 有
    B. 没有
    C. 打算参加

二、学习习惯、态度和风格

10. 你有课前预习的习惯吗?
    A. 经常有
    B. 偶尔有
    C. 几乎没有
11. 你有课后及时巩固的习惯吗?
    A. 经常有
    B. 偶尔有
    C. 几乎没有
12. 你上课会经常带着问题去听吗?
    A. 经常有
    B. 偶尔有
    C. 几乎没有
13. 上课遇到听不懂的地方,怎么办?
    A. 及时举手提问
    B. 算了,没弄懂先跳过去,课后问教师同学
    C. 不问了,就听只任之,过去了
    D. 干脆干其他事,开小差
14. 课后遇到难题,怎么办?
    A. 查资料,想方设法弄懂
    B. 和同学讨论
    C. 自己苦思冥想
    D. 不解决
15. 教师布置的作业会独立、及时完成吗?
    A. 会的
    B. 偶尔不会
    C. 经常不会
    D. 绝不会
16. 对学习抱何态度?
    A. 想把它学好并努力
    B. 想把它学好,但太难了就放弃
    C. 无所谓
    D. 通过考试就行

三、教师授课风格和方式

17. 你喜欢什么样的上课方式?
    A. 教师讲授
    B. 分组讨论
    C. 同学自己演示或表演
    D. 实际操作

E. 其他(请列出：　　　)　　　　F. 都不喜欢

18. 你在课堂上能主动参与到教师组织的活动中吗？
    A. 常常很主动　　B. 一般　　　　C. 较少　　　　D. 从不
19. 你希望教师在教与学方面应该做些什么？
    A. 教师在课堂上多分享一些学科的最新进展或扩展的知识
    B. 按照课本内容授课
    C. 只讲与考试相关的内容，其他的不愿意听
    D. 无所谓
20. 你喜欢的教师是？
    A. 学养深厚的　　B. 风趣的　　　　C. 漂亮的　　　　D. 无所谓
21. 你希望本门课程的考试方式是？
    A. 开卷考(较难)　　　　　　　　B. 闭卷考(较容易)
    C. 写长篇综述　　　　　　　　　D. 其他(请写出)

谢谢你的参与！

课 后 问 卷

专业　　　　　班级　　　　　性别

同学们，大家好！此问卷是为了解同学们的学习状况和需求，不会影响考试成绩，请如实填写。每一问题后均有若干选项，请在符合自己情况的选项前打勾，相容性的选项可多选。

一、对课程的掌握和感受

1. 学习了本课程后，你对其内容掌握程度是？
   A. 掌握得很好　　　　　　　　　B. 掌握了大部分
   C. 掌握了一些基本的　　　　　　D. 完全没有掌握
2. 学习这门课程后，你对该课程内容的感受是？
   A. 非常感兴趣　　　　　　　　　B. 有意思，还行
   C. 无所谓　　　　　　　　　　　D. 不感兴趣
3. 你觉得循证医学对临床实践的重要程度是？
   A. 非常重要　　　　　　　　　　B. 重要
   C. 不重要　　　　　　　　　　　D. 不知道，不好说

4. 你觉得你在该门课上学到的最重要的内容是?(可以多选)

　　A. 任何决策都要循证的思想　　　　B. 证据的分级思想和分级方法

　　C. 证据检索的方法　　　　　　　　D. 临床文献的阅读方法

　　E. 临床研究的评价方法

　　F. 一些统计指标(如 RR 值)的计算方法

　　G. Meta 分析的制作方法

　　H. 提供证据的系统(如临床指南、Cochrane Library)

　　I. 其他(请列出:　　)

5. 你觉得你在这门课上学到的会对你将来的工作和学习有用吗?

　　A. 非常有用　　　　B. 应该有用　　　　C. 没有什么用　　D. 不知道

6. 你觉得这门课程难度如何?

　　A. 非常难　　　　　B. 有些难　　　　　C. 不难　　　　　D. 太简单了

7. 你在这门课程上所花的精力如何?

　　A. 花了大量精力　　B. 花了一些精力　　C. 完全不花精力

8. 你参加过或正在参加科研课题吗?

　　A. 有　　　　　　　B. 没有　　　　　　C. 打算参加

二、教师授课风格和方式

9. 你喜欢这门课的哪个环节?(可多选)

　　A. 教师讲授　　　　　　　　　　　B. TPS

　　C. 头脑风暴　　　　　　　　　　　D. 实际操作

　　E. 小组讨论和任务　　　　　　　　F. 个人作业

　　G 其他(请列出:　　　　)　　　　H. 都不喜欢

10. 你在本门课堂上能主动参与到教师组织的活动中吗?

　　A. 常常很主动　　B. 一般　　　　　C. 较少　　　　　D. 从不

11. 你觉得教师在本门课程中采用的案例有意思吗?

　　A. 非常有意思　　B. 有意思,还行　　C. 无所谓　　　　D. 没意思

12. 你觉得教师在教学哪些方面做得比较好?(可多选)

　　A. 讲授逻辑　　　　　　　　　　　B. 时间掌控

　　C. 与同学互动　　　　　　　　　　D. 分享心得

　　E. 知识扩展　　　　　　　　　　　F. 其他(请列出:　　　　)

13. 你觉得本门课程的成绩组成合理吗?(考勤+平时作业+期中成绩+期末成绩)

　　A. 非常合理　　　　　　　　　　　B. 还行

　　C. 不合理　　　　　　　　　　　　D. 我希望是另一种(请列出:　　　　)

14. 你对本门课程教师评价是?（请按 5-1 之状况评价，5：完全同意，4：同意
    3：尚可 2：不同意 1：完全不同意）

    A. 学养丰厚（5   4   3   2   1）

    B. 风趣幽默（5   4   3   2   1）

    C. 气质高雅（5   4   3   2   1）

    D. 和蔼亲切（5   4   3   2   1）

    E. 逻辑清晰（5   4   3   2   1）

    F. 其他（请列出并评分：   ）

15. 关于课程，如你有其他的建议或意见，请列出：

谢谢你的参与！

Appendix Ⅰ

Questionnaires

Questionnaire Before Class

Major   Class   Gender

Hello, everyone! This questionnaire is to understand your learning situation and needs, and it will not impact your final scores. Please fill in it truthfully. There are several options for each question. Please tick the option which is fit for you, you can multiselect if the choices are compatible.

I. Understanding of the course

1. Have you previewed the content before you learn it?
   A. Yes.   B. No.
2. Are you interested in this course while knowing its name?
   A. Very interested.   B. Interested a little bit.
   C. Doesn't matter.   D. Not interested.
3. How much do you know about evidence-based medicine?
   A. Very much.   B. A little bit.
   C. Have heard about it.   D. Never heard about it.
4. When it comes to "evidence-based medicine", what do you think of it?
   A. Looking up articles.
   B. Meta-analysis and RCT.
   C. Making clinical decision based on evidence.
   D. Nothing.
5. Do you think evidence-based medicine will be useful for your future work and study?
   A. Vey useful.   B. Should be useful.
   C. There's nothing to do with it. D. Don't know.

6. Epidemiology deals with?

    A. Diagnosis and treatment of infectious disease.

    B. Diagnosis and treatment of Epidemic disease.

    C. Distribution and determinants of disease and health situation in specific population.

    D. I don't know.

7. How much do you the statistical knowledge?

    A. Very much.   B. A little.

    C. Have heard about it.   D. Never heard about it.

8. How much do you know literature retrieval knowledge and skills?

    A. Very much, I can acquire any literature I need.

    B. Just ok.

    C. Have forgotten everything I learnt about it.

    D. Never heard about it.

9. Have you ever been participated or are you participating in a scientific research project?

    A. Yes.   B. No.   C. Intend to.

II. Learning habits, attitudes and styles

10. Do you have the habit of previewing before class?

    A. Usually.

    B. Occasionally.

    C. Few.

11. Do you have the habit of reviewing after class?

    A. Usually.

    B. Occasionally.

    C. Few.

12. Do you listen to the teacher with questions?

    A. Usually.

    B. Occasionally.

    C. Few.

13. What would you do when you cannot understand the teacher?

    A. Raise hands in time to ask questions.

    B. Ask the teacher or classmates after class.

    C. Never ask.

    D. Do other unrelated things instead of listening.

14. What would you do when you come across difficulties in study after class?

    A. Try to understand in all ways.　B. Discuss them with classmates.

    C. Think it myself.　　　　　　　D. Never mind.

15. Would you finish the homework independently and in time?

    A. Of course.　　　　　　　　　B. Occasionally not.

    C. Usually not.　　　　　　　　　D. Never.

16. What is your attitude towards learning?

    A. I try my best to learn it.　　B. I quit if it is too hard.

    C. Never mind.　　　　　　　　　D. I just want to pass the exam.

III. Teachers' teaching styles and methods

17. What kind of teaching style do you like? (can be multiple choice)

    A. lecture

    B. TPS

    C. group discussion or working

    D. demonstrating by us students

    E. operating by ourselves

    F. others (please list:　　)

    G. I like none of them.

18. Would you participate in the activities which teacher organized in class?

    A. Usually.　　　　　　　　　　B. Sometimes.

    C. Few times.　　　　　　　　　D. never.

19. What do you want the teacher to do in teaching?

    A. The teacher shares the latest progress or other expanded knowledge.

    B. Teaching according to the contents of the textbook.

    C. Just talk about the content related to the exam; I have no willing to listen to other things unrelated to the final exam.

    D. Don't mind.

20. Which kind of teacher do you like?

    A. Knowledgeable.　　　　　　　B. Funny.

    C. Pretty.　　　　　　　　　　　D. Don't mind.

21. Which kind of exam do you like in this course?

A. Open-book exam (hard).   B. close-book examination (easy).
C. Writing a review.   D. Others (please list:).

Thank you for your participation!

Questionnaire After Class

Major   Class   Gender

Hello, everyone! This questionnaire is to understand your learning situation and needs, and it will not impact your final scores, please fill in it truthfully. There are several options for each question. Please tick the option which is fit for you. You can do multiselect if the choices are compatible.

I. Understanding of the course

1. How much do you master the content after learning the course?
   A. Very well.   B. Most of it.
   C. Mastered some of the basics. D. Definitely nothing.
2. How do you feel about this course after learning?
   A. I'm interested very much.   B. Not bad.
   C. I don't mind.   D. I'm not interested.
3. How important do you think is evidence-based medicine to clinical practice?
   A. Very important.   B. Important.
   C. Not important.   D. Hard to say.
4. What is the most important thing you think you learned in this course? (multiple choices are allowed)
   A. Any decision-making should be based on evidence.
   B. The thought and method of grading evidence.
   C. Methods of evidence retrieval.
   D. How to read a clinical literature.
   E. Methods of appraising a clinical research.
   F. How to calculate some statistical indicators, such as RR.
   G. Methodology of producing Meta-analysis.

H. Systems providing evidence（such as clinical guidelines，Cochrane Library）.

I. Other（please list：　）

5. Do you think what you learned in this class will be useful for your future work and study?

A. Very useful.　　　　　　　B. Should be useful.

C. Not useful.　　　　　　　D. I don't know.

6. How difficult do you think of this course?

A Very difficult.　　　　　　B. A little difficult.

C. It's not hard.　　　　　　D. It's too easy.

7. How much effort do you spend on this course?

A. A lot.　　　B. Some.　　　C. Completely no.

8. Have you ever been participated or are you participating in a scientific research project?

A. Yes.　　　B. No.　　　C. Intend to.

II. Teachers' teaching styles and methods

9. Which part of the course do you like?（multiple choices are allowed）

A. the lectures teacher gave　　B. TPS

C. brainstorming　　　　　　D. practical operation

E. group discussion and task　F. personal assignments

G. think break　　　　　　　H. other interactions（please list：　）

I. none

10. Have you participated in the activities or interactions which teacher organized in class?

A. Usually.　B. Sometimes.　C. Few times.　D. Never.

11. Do you think the teacher's cases in this course are interesting?

A. Most of them are very interesting.

B. They are ok.

C. I don't mind.

D. Most of them are not interesting.

12. Which part do you think the teacher did well in teaching?

（multiple choices are allowed）

A. logic stating part

     B. time-control during the class

     C. interactions

     D. sharing insights

     E. extension of knowledge

     F. others (please list:　　)

13. Do you think the composition of the final score is reasonable? (attendance + homework + interim exam + final exam)

     A. Very reasonable.

     B. Ok.

     C. Unreasonable.

     D. I hope to be another (please list:　　).

14. What is your evaluation of the teacher group? (The meanings of the numbers are following. 5: totally agree with it; 4: agree with it; 3: ok; 2: do not agree with it; 1: totally disagree with it.)

     A. knowledgeable (5　4　3　2　1)

     B. with humor (5　4　3　2　1)

     C. elegant (5　4　3　2　1)

     D. kind (5　4　3　2　1)

     E. clear logic (5　4　3　2　1)

     F. others (please list and score:　　)

15. If you have other suggestions or comments, please list:

Thank you for your participation!

KWL 表

姓名_____ 日期_____

　　选择一个你感兴趣的研究主题。在第一栏写下关于这个主题你已经知道的内容。在第二栏写下关于这个主题你想知道的内容。当你完成研究任务后,在第三栏写下你学到的内容。

我已经知道的	我想知道的	我学到的

KWL chart

Name：_____ Date：_____

Select a topic you want to research. In the first column, write down what you already know about the topic. In the second column, write down what you want to know about the topic. After you have completed your research, write down what you learned in the third column.

What I Know	What I Want to Know	What I Learned